Acclaim for Harry Glorikian's

THE FUTURE YOU

The Future You is a concise and relatable synthesis of the bleeding edge of biomedical research. If you feel excitement and wonder from reading the latest news headlines of sci-fi–like breakthroughs in artificial intelligences and biomedicine, yet find yourself wondering, 'What does this mean for me?', then you will find no better guide than *The Future You*. In the spirit of the enduring William Gibson quote, 'The future is here—it's just not evenly distributed,' *The Future You* astonishes readers with stories from the frontlines of biomedical innovation happening today while providing relatable and actionable information on how you can take action in your own daily life to anticipate and participate in the coming biomedical revolution.

—Joel Dudley, PhD, Chief Scientific Officer, Tempus Labs, Inc.

AI and technology are disrupting healthcare at an unprecedented rate, reshaping how we treat and address disease. Author Harry Glorikian is able to distill complex biomedical science from the experts into thoughtful explanations and insights on how readers can benefit from these advancements in their own health and wellness journeys. *The Future You* examines what is possible from leading healthcare researchers and practitioners as they work to discover better ways to treat patients and improve lives.

—Andrew Radin, CEO, Aria Pharmaceuticals

The Future You provides a glimpse into the fascinating and unique dimensions of medical and biomedical research in healthcare. As with Stephen Hawkings and his predicted breakthroughs in astrophysics, AI will continue to reveal deeper insights into the way the body works and the new strategies we need to adopt to lead healthy lives. Since becoming a doctor in biomedical sciences and a clinician, I've discovered that there is more that we don't know than answers to what we do know. Every human and every other living thing on this beautiful planet shares this trait. As a patient with a rare disease who battles multiple sclerosis–like and Parkinson's-like symptoms, my life so far confirms my observation that we need to understand the *making of us*.

In light of the advances in genomics, artificial intelligence, and microbiome research discussed in *The Future You*, I am more optimistic that the future will bring a lot of hope to patients such as myself. With a focus on that future, this book will serve as an invaluable primer for patients, physicians, healthcare innovators, investors, and the general public. A deep insight into healthcare innovation provided in *The Future You* is the ultimate blessing any reader will reach based on Hippocrates' declaration: "Health is the greatest blessing in life."

It is time to know *you* as a supreme being, so that you can become the most incredible version of yourself possible.

—*Dr Kamala Maddali, President, Health Collaborations, a Rare Disease Patient and Healthcare Changemaker*

In the future we'll see a shift from short-term sick care to prioritizing preventive long-term healthcare. Integrating AI, data, and technology into the industry is the only way to get there. Harry Glorikian's analysis of the smart medicine movement in *The Future You* is the blueprint to how we can live better, healthier lives.

—*Harpreet Singh Rai, CEO, Oura*

It's inevitable that the practice of medicine is on the verge of a quantified and intelligent revolution. Just as in other industries before it, healthcare and medicine will be more personalized and hopefully proactive. In some cases, medical care will be a completely digital experience. *The Future You* brings this vision to life and details the tangible progress being made in traditional medicines, medical devices, healthcare companies, inventive startups, and technology giants. It's a must-read not just for fans of the "digital health" industry, but for all individuals interested in a future where medicine is made and delivered uniquely "for me and powered uniquely by me and my data."

—*Christine Lemke, Co-CEO and Co-founder, Evidation*

THE FUTURE YOU

How Artificial Intelligence Can Help You Get Healthier, Stress Less, and Live Longer

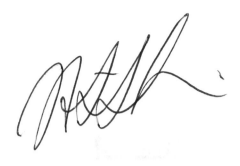

THE FUTURE YOU

How Artificial Intelligence Can Help You Get Healthier, Stress Less, and Live Longer

HARRY GLORIKIAN

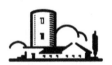

Brick Tower Press
New York

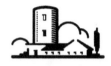

Brick Tower Press
Manhanset House
Dering Harbor, New York 11965-0342
bricktower@aol.com
www.BrickTowerPress.com

Library of Congress Cataloging-in-Publication Data
The Future You: How Artificial Intelligence Can Help You Get Healthier, Stress Less, and Live Longer
Glorikian, Harry

p. cm.
1. COMPUTERS—Intelligence (AI) & Semantics
2. MEDICAL—Health Policy 3. MEDICAL—Medical History & Records 4. MEDICAL—Physician & Patient
I. Title
Includes references

ISBN: 978–1–883283–82–7, Trade Paper
978-1-883283-83-4, Hardcover
First Edition October 2021

ACKNOWLEDGMENTS

The support of the following individuals is greatly appreciated:

Kevin Banks, Owner/Art Director
Claymore Design

John T. Colby Jr., Publisher
Brick Tower Press

Dr. Robert Green, MD, MPH, Professor/Geneticist
Harvard Medical School
Brigham and Women's Hospital
Broad Institute

Jennifer Malinowski, MS, PhD, Senior Methodologist
American College of Medical Genetics and Genomics
(*The greatest partner in brainstorming my ideas and helping me
shape them through constructive dialogue and debate*)

Alan Morell, Chairman/Chief Executive Officer
Creative Management Agency

Wade Roush, Journalist
Soonish podcast

Mike Slizewski, Editor
Brick Tower Press

DEDICATION

I'd first like to thank my wife, Katrina, who has always supported me in all my adventures. I would also like to thank my mother, Elizabeth Glorikian (1927-2012), for always being my greatest cheerleader.

TABLE OF CONTENTS

FOREWORD

By Dr. Bob Arnot

The doctor is in your device.

The late John McCarthy coined the term "artificial intelligence"—AI, for short—for a talk he gave at a now legendary Dartmouth conference in 1956, where he predicted that " ... every aspect of learning or feature of intelligence can, in principle, be described so accurately that you can create a machine that simulates them." Known as "the father of artificial intelligence," McCarthy dedicated his long life to AI research—but even he would be surprised at how far the field has come in recent years.

So what exactly is artificial intelligence? In the computer science world, it describes a device—whether digital computer or computer-controlled robot or the like—that is able to improve its own performance. A machine that teaches itself to think, to learn on its own.

AI is all around us. Self-driving cars. Smart personal assistants—think Siri, Cortana, or Google Now— or Alexa, Amazon's cloud-based voice service that is available on literally hundreds of millions of devices. Voice-to-text. Manufacturing robots. Facial recognition software. Security surveillance. Automated financial investing and social media monitoring. Smart homes that control themselves when their owners are out of town. The list is endless.

All of the above make life *easier* for us. But in this new book by *Moneyball Medicine* investor/author/podcaster Harry Glorikian, the spotlight is on how AI can (and will, and in many cases already does) make us *healthier*.

Do you have a smartphone and a wearable device, such as an Apple Watch or a Fitbit? Most likely yes, right? Well, then, as Glorikian tells us, there are already numerous apps available for download that " ... can also continuously monitor temperature, calorie intake, blood glucose, menstruation cycle, respiration rate, stress levels, brain waves, or just about any other aspect of physical and mental health you want." They identify areas where improvement is needed, and tell us *how* to improve our health in those areas.

Meanwhile, AI (and big data) research is enabling medical practitioners to predict debilitating diseases years in advance, thereby (hopefully) improving the odds of mitigating some of the devastating effects of those diseases through the field of genetics, which also relies strongly on AI. It can help address and ultimately prevent pandemics. It enables doctors to diagnose more quickly and accurately. It provides remote medical assistance to those who are unable for whatever reason to receive that assistance in person.

(On a side note, while this book doesn't directly consider it, global health is an issue that is dear to my heart. I have traveled the world as a doctor and medical journalist. I also have an abiding commitment to humanitarian causes, because in the course of my travels, I have witnessed—and reported on—countless examples of needless pain and suffering. Rampant diseases and epidemics that flourish because people don't have access to the kind of medical treatment that is at our fingertips. Imagine how the issues Glorikian addresses here will ultimately affect the rest of the world as the technology expands—in much the same way that we saw cell phones leapfrogging throughout the world—and how that can change healthcare in different parts of the world.)

I am also a lifelong athlete—a fitness enthusiast, if you will. And I can tell you from that lifetime of experience that feeling good feels … well, really good. Taking care of yourself should be your number-one priority—for you, for your family, friends, and community, and frankly, for the planet. AI is making this easier, and doing so at an exponential rate, as *The Future You* so aptly illustrates.

So—how can this book change your perspective and approach to your own health and well-being? The author provides a perfect personal example: he identified his own previously undiagnosed sleep apnea—he was alerted to it by his Apple Watch! And that same device helps him monitor and control that condition.

The old saying, "You have to be your own doctor," has always been true, but it has never before been more within our reach. We'll always need doctors, of course—I don't foresee my colleagues and I populating the unemployment lines as a result of these medical advances (at least not the ones who embrace this rapidly developing technology).

And as a doctor, I have a recommendation. When you finish reading this book, don't put it back on the shelf. Make it the centerpiece of your coffee table, and be sure to share it wherever and whenever possible. It can make all the difference in the quality of your life. Glorikian not only shows us the possibilities, but just how close we are to "the future us." We're almost there!

The doctor is in your device, indeed.

—Bob Arnot, MD, is the New York Times *bestselling author of fourteen books on nutrition and health. He has been a medical correspondent for* NBC Nightly News, Dateline NBC, 60 Minutes, *and* CBS This Morning. *He is the author of courses on* Artificial Intelligence and Medicine, Deep Learning and Healthcare, *and* Machine Learning and Healthcare *(*https://www.devry.edu/online-programs/courses/deep-learning-in-medicine.html*), and is the former host of the* Dr. Danger *reality TV series. An avid competitor who has represented the US in eight world championships in stand up surfing, Nordic ski racing (including at the World Masters Nationals in Norway), and ski mountaineering racing (or Skimo—now an Olympic sport, he competed for the US at the World Winter Games in Austria), Dr. Arnot lives in Palm Beach, Florida, and Vermont.*

INTRODUCTION

EVERYTHING YOU KNOW ABOUT YOUR HEALTH IS GOING TO CHANGE

If you can't measure something, you can't understand it. If you can't understand it, you can't control it. If you can't control it, you can't improve it."—H. James Harrington, PhD, former IBM quality expert and businessman

"In God we trust, all others bring data."—W. Edwards Deming, engineer and statistician

New York City. The epicenter of the coronavirus crisis in the US.

For millions living in urban areas, it's not a difficult place or time to imagine, since the same panic played out on city streets all over the world.

But there you are, ringed in with millions of others on the two-mile-wide island of Manhattan. The virus is raging through the Big Apple, sickening thousands in seemingly random fashion. Some get violently sick; others show only mild symptoms or nothing at all. Doctors say asymptomatic patients are spreading the illness, but there's no way to know who might fall ill, when, or where.

As the city's death count climbs, overwhelming morgues and funeral homes, you hope that you and those in your immediate household don't come into contact with an infected person—or contract the virus from a surface where it's silently been festering for days. No one knows how it spreads or how to keep themselves safe from the disease. In the absence of widespread testing, your only option, it seems, is to sit, wait, and take every precaution against a contagion that's infecting even the most vigilant. It's as if the 2011 film *Contagion* has become a nightmarish reality.

This kind of fear and anxiety was playing out in apartments and townhomes across New York City during the coronavirus crisis. While nothing can take away the tragedy and loss of lives that COVID-19 wrought upon the US's biggest city—and the world at large—I can't help but wonder how things might have been different if more people knew how products enabled by artificial intelligence (AI), many of which already exist, could have helped them to learn they may have had COVID-19 before they were symptomatic, allowing them to get tested, quarantine, and minimize the spread of the illness. Devices that could be used to monitor their health status at home, with the information sent directly to their doctors, so that doctors could identify which patients were getting better on their own, and who needed medical intervention.

An app called Coughvid, for example, was developed within weeks of the first deaths from the virus in the US to predict the presence of COVID-19 from the sound of a cough alone. Other apps followed, many looking to diagnose, prevent, or monitor symptoms of the virus, regardless of where you live, your access to testing, and whether or when you can see a doctor. Researchers at the University of California, San Francisco used the Oura Ring for its TemPredict Study, finding that patterns in the data from Oura users predicted onset of fever and other symptoms, prompting users to get tested for COVID-19. Front-line healthcare workers at Mount Sinai Hospital participated in the Warrior Watch study that uses an Apple Watch to evaluate how they were handling the effects of COVID-19. Researchers there found that they were able to uncover patterns in participants' data that predicted a positive COVID-19 diagnosis up to a week before laboratory tests. Imagine how earlier knowledge about your health from these devices and wearables, much like a tornado siren or earthquake or tsunami alarm alert folks in an area to take cover, your phone or app could tell you to shelter in place, remind you to ask a friend to bring you some soup and tissues (masked of course), and schedule a drive-through testing appointment for confirmation.

These are just a few of the countless Artificial Intelligence (AI)-enabled tools, gadgets, and gizmos that are changing everything we know about our healthcare. AI and big data are combining in incredible ways to make predictions about patient outcomes that are oftentimes more accurate than what's possible with the human eye or hand. Here's what AI and big data are already accomplishing or aiming to accomplish in healthcare:

- Identifying early onset of diseases like cancer years before patients are diagnosed
- Alerting patients when they're sick before they develop symptoms
- Discovering new cures for previously untreatable conditions
- Finding the right therapy at the right time for the right patient
- Making sure newborn babies will be healthy before they're born
- Tailor-fitting your diet to your body type to help you lose weight
- Creating an exercise regimen personalized to your individual fitness
- Helping you stress less and sleep more

In short, the applications are endless, and the impacts are far-reaching. There's not a person among us who isn't going to feel the effects of this AI revolution, and it's going to utterly transform the healthcare system as we know it today.

This isn't an oversell. And I'm not trying to wiggle buzzwords like "artificial intelligence" and "big data" into areas they don't belong. I know AI and big data will upend healthcare, because they already are.

How to Beat Vegas, Be a Better Tour Guide, and Win the World Series

To get to the present, let's start with the past and a story about the power of predictive analytics—a term that would change my personal perspective and eventually transform medicine.

The year is 1984. The place is San Francisco. I'm nineteen years old. This is when I start to work for the man who will be my first real boss and mentor. He runs a computer education business, and I'm his all-around office assistant, helping him assemble manuals, book flights for teachers to in-person classes (this was before the Internet age and online learning), and ship all necessary instruction materials. It's not just my first office job, but also my first exposure to computers. Under his tutelage, I learn how to assemble PCs and get the systems up and running.

I also learn something else that challenges my teenage brain. My boss is brilliant and thinks about the world in a new and different way. I always assumed he made his money as a computer coach. While he did earn a nice living from his education business, he didn't make all of his money teaching entrepreneurs how to turn a PC on and off.

Instead, my boss invented a kind of computer that could help predict the winning bet on roulette and other games of chance. The system, which he and his friends created, could calculate the speed at which a particular roulette ball orbited around a roulette wheel based on a mathematical formula, or algorithm, which was similar to the kinds of math used by NASA to land rockets on the moon. The math didn't work out every time, but it gave him a 44 percent advantage in a game with one of the worst odds in the house. This meant that if he let an initial bet of $100 ride fifty times over the course of one hour, he'd make $2,200. That was a pretty darn good hourly rate in the 1970s when he first started playing, and I'd say it's still a good rate today, at $17,600 per day, assuming an eight-hour workday.

For me, the moral of the story at the time wasn't to quit college and create a computer that would turn me into a professional gambler overnight. Instead, the point was the profound outcomes you could achieve using smart data and a little bit of math. It illustrated statistics and probability at its best and was my first real brush with predictive analytics—the art of using data (and complex mathematical formulas) to establish a pattern to predict an outcome. Nineteen-year-old me wasn't thinking about how this might upend major industries in the future, but the concept of predictive analytics was planted in my brain, where it was destined to flourish, it turns out, for years to come.

Flash forward to 1999 and the Boston suburbs, where I now live with my wife and two children. I never thought I'd trade Silicon Valley for the East Coast hotbed of biotech, but there I am, in the heart of the republic—where the first shots of the Revolutionary War were fired—and I love it. By this point, I'd spent a number of years in biotech, and Boston felt like home.

At the time, I was working for Applied Biosystems (ABI) in nearby Framingham, Massachusetts. The company was making technical platforms to assist scientists with the Human Genome Project, a $3 billion, thirteen-year international effort to sequence the whole human genome, which they finally did in 2003. My day-to-day job exposed me to the world of DNA and a new concept at the time called bioinformatics, which combines biology and information technology. Big data and analytics were at the forefront of my thoughts—data and genomics danced together in my dreams at night. It was one of the most enjoyable times of my career. ABI was sometimes said to stand for Arrogance Beyond Imagination, but I knew we were changing the world.

On a sun-washed day in the fall of 1999, I was driving my sister and brother-in-law, who were in town from the Bay Area, through the birthplace of our country's freedom, Concord, Massachusetts. Everyone was chatting, but I was concentrating in order to play tour guide. The Boston suburbs are literally littered with historic sites, so if I wanted to chime in on a conversation my passengers were having (for example, on how San Francisco's Sunset District had changed since I lived there as a kid), we'd go hurtling past Walden Pond, home of Henry David Thoreau, without anyone getting a whiff of that storied "tonic of wildness." Through it all, I was also paying attention to every little sign sticking out of the ground, because this was 1999, long before GPS became the tool that everyone takes for granted today. I could either play tour guide or catch up with family and friends as we drove around Boston—it was just too hard to do both at the same time.

This sort of trip was always frustrating. There were dozens of historical sites I wanted to show my family, including restaurants, businesses, and other personal points of interest, but instead, I was constantly pulling over to consult my historical guidebook and AAA Road Atlas. How could mankind be on the edge of mapping out the human genome, but we couldn't use the same technology in an interactive way to map out our own world?

As I was driving, an idea popped into my head. I went home and started researching. Several months later, I filed my first patent for position-related services that would use GPS data, along with your speed, direction, and time, to alert you to when you were approaching a historical site, contemporary landmark, favorite restaurant, or other important place. The more you used my AI-enabled device—that is, the more data it collected on your habits, which restaurants you liked, whether you preferred Civil War or Civil Rights history—the more my device would be able to "learn" what you liked.

At the time, industries tended to be fairly siloed, and it was difficult for a life sciences guy to break into what was then the sole world of telecom. The two fields just couldn't comprehend how one could have meaningful insight for the other—and my idea didn't go far. Today, the idea of combining GPS with historical and current information that personalizes the application based on personal preferences not only seems obvious, it's a multibillion-dollar industry called "location-based services," which includes Waze and Google Maps.

Fast-forward ten years to 2011. This is when the appeal of data and predictive analytics really hits its stride, thanks to the movie *Moneyball*, with Brad Pitt and Jonah Hill. *Moneyball*, based on the best-selling book by Michael Lewis, doesn't have anything to do with the AI that we utilize today—there's no smart computer that "learns" what baseball coaches need or want in a new player. Instead, that work is done by the brains of Oakland A's general manager Billy Beane and his Ivy League–educated assistant manager, Peter Brand, who convinces Beane to use sabermetrics—baseball-specific statistics—to recruit new players.

Faced with a budget that won't let the A's even wink at a high-talent player, Beane applies Brand's sabermetrics to sign a ragtag bunch of injured, aging, obscure, or otherwise seemingly undesirable recruits. His choices anger the A's head scout and manager to the point where it looks like Beane may lose his job. But he believes in the data and the possibility that the odd-shaped cogs of players he's chosen will come together into one well-oiled machine, even if neither Beane nor Brand can see it at the time. As the movie progresses, this is exactly what happens, as Beane and Brand's unconventional choices turn into a hit team that eventually wins the 2002 World Series.

Moneyball's real-life success story sent sports teams and companies scrambling to apply the "moneyball" methodology to nearly every sports franchise and business. The movie's commercial success also led me to believe the world was ready to see how the same methodology was already being used in healthcare. The government had recently mandated that hospitals and doctors' offices needed to transfer their patients' paper files to electronic health records, which would only speed the adoption of predictive analytics in medicine. In 2013, I started writing *Moneyball Medicine*, a book I published several years later that shows how data-driven technology is disrupting healthcare and life sciences.

Predicting outcomes becomes easier when you don't have to rely on human brains like Billy Beane's and Peter Brand's, but you can filter that information instead through a system that simulates human intelligence to forecast just about anything you want it to. For the past few years, I've watched with excitement as AI and big data have made more and more predictions about our lives, with startling accuracy, as the data has grown larger and the computers that use it faster and smarter.

To see how AI, big data, and predictive analytics impact our everyday lives, all you need to do is spend a few minutes surfing the website of one of the most valuable companies in the world: Amazon. The online retailer has more data about you and its millions of other customers than you can fathom. Not only does it log everything you click, buy, or place in your shopping cart, Amazon also tracks census information, shipping addresses (which can indicate income level), returns, feedback, reviews, and even photos snapped using its virtual assistant, Alexa. Amazon then crunches all this data to sell you more stuff. The retail giant does this by using AI-enabled computers that "learn" what you like.

For example, its algorithms send you a suggestion for new underwear because you've clicked, carted, or bought other items like cologne, shaving razors, and protein powder. Based on what other consumers have purchased after clicking, carting, or buying these same items, Amazon assumes you're about to improve your love life.

Amazon's supercomputers do all this completely independent of human interference—that is, there is no bleary-eyed worker inside Amazon's HQ cuing up product suggestions for its bazillion customers. This is what makes

AI "intelligent"—the technology makes decisions independent of the human brain that created it.

Moneyball's Effect on Medicine: Predicting a Healthier You

What happens when you apply the trifecta of AI, big data, and predictive analytics to healthcare?

You get something more valuable than a better baseball team, new underwear on Amazon, or even a fistful of Vegas chips—you get the potential to prevent disease, optimize your health, and even increase what Michael Geer, cofounder and chief strategy officer of Humanity Health, calls your healthspan: the number of years of healthy, functioning life. You might even find that healthcare becomes, in some ways, less expensive: we're getting the right drug to the right person at the right time, and with less trial and error than expensive medications that don't work. We find the cancer earlier when treatment is less invasive and less costly. We identify the very earliest stages of diabetes before you need lifelong insulin or other medication, and we help you lose weight, exercise more efficiently, and eat healthier.

While medicine has been slow to adopt AI and big data—there's more to lose when you forecast whether a patient will get cancer than whether a Netflix user will want to watch the new season of *Ozark*—the trifecta is already transforming healthcare in breathtaking ways.

AI, for example, is being used in intensive care units (ICUs) to alert doctors when a patient might have a heart attack or other life-threatening event before the event occurs. How? The AI-enabled device is fed thousands of past patient records to "learn" which vital signs most often preempt a heart attack. The device then monitors the vitals of current ICU patients. If it notices Judy in Room 331 has signs similar to those of past heart-attack patients, the device will signal a doctor to examine Judy or intervene immediately before her likely heart attack occurs. On the other hand, the AI system could also identify when patients have improved and are ready for care at a less-intensive level, may be ready to move out of the ICU into a general care ward, or reduce a patient's medication. The actual nuts and bolts of the AI system are more complicated, but this is basically how it works.

Here's another example that might hit closer to home—it certainly hit closer to my home. Recently, I downloaded Apple's free Cardiogram app, which monitors your heart-rate activity using data from an Apple Watch or Fitbit. Both wrist devices have a heart-rate sensor that can record pulse continuously while also tracking sleep and physical activity and feeding all this information back to Cardiogram.

I hadn't been using Cardiogram for more than a few months when the app flashed a warning sign. "Do you have sleep apnea?" Cardiogram wanted to know. I was shocked and intrigued. I had been diagnosed a few years earlier with the disorder, which can cause your airway to close at night, interrupting normal breathing and increasing the risk of heart problems and neurological disease. When I told Cardiogram I did, the app wanted to know if I was being treated for the condition. Cardiogram wanted to further hone its data on me, improving its collective information bank and ability to predict individual outcome.

Cardiogram isn't just knowledgeable on sleep disorders. Since its launch in 2016, the app has been credited with saving lives by alerting users to heart irregularities that can cause stroke and other fatal events with 97 percent accuracy.

Your smartphone and the apps you download, either individually or combined with a wearable device, can also continuously monitor temperature, calorie intake, blood glucose, menstruation cycle, respiration rate, stress levels, brain waves, or just about any other aspect of physical and mental health you want. Specific apps then use this information to suggest how you can improve your diet, sleep, sex life, body mass index, exercise, mood, cognitive health, and more. The technology is evolving to tell you exactly how many hours of sleep you need, whether a three-mile jog or thirty-minute weight workout would be more beneficial to your body type, and if a keto diet or a calorie-controlled plan would help you lose the most weight in the least amount of time.

Outside the home, doctors and researchers are using AI and big data to identify whether a patient might develop a disease like cancer or Alzheimer's years before symptoms show. Data-driven technology is also helping physicians predict whether expecting parents will have a healthy baby or whether a newborn might develop a disease that could be thwarted in the child's early years. AI and big data are helping researchers develop new drugs for cancer and rare diseases. The field is also rapidly advancing to try to predict and prevent another pandemic like the COVID-19 before it kills thousands and cripples the world economy.

Data-driven technology in healthcare is here—and it's already saving lives. Throughout this book, you'll learn the specific ways in which AI and big data are preventing disease, finding new treatments, tailor-fitting drugs to treat individuals, helping people live longer, warding off global outbreaks, and teaching us all how to stress less, get leaner, and be healthier and happier. And we're only at the beginning …

How Data-driven Technology Saves Time, Money, and Lives

The scenarios I'm going to describe in this book don't just apply to someone with a rare condition or who is seriously ill—these are examples of how everyone can take advantage of AI and data analytics to stay healthy, get diagnosed more quickly, and sometimes, save on healthcare costs.

A sixty-five-year-old Houston man began to feel his heart race as he was winding down for the night.

Typically, our heart rates slow down a bit as we get ready for bed and fall asleep. Anthony Purser's heart was doing the opposite. Like most of us would, Purser saw his doctor, but because his heart rate was fine during the day, his doctor couldn't immediately pinpoint the cause. Even once his heart rate became more erratic during the day, it wasn't something that was apparent during doctor visits—but his cardiologist had an idea what was behind Purser's racing heartbeat and how to catch it in the act.

Purser's doctor suspected the man had atrial fibrillation, a serious medical condition that can, if untreated, lead to stroke or heart failure. He recommended the Houston man wear an Apple Watch with a built-in electrocardiogram (ECG or EKG) function, so he could check it several times during the day, and importantly, when he was feeling his heart racing. After a few weeks of using his smartwatch to monitor his heart, Purser downloaded the data and took it to his cardiology appointment, allowing the doctor to officially diagnose the atrial fibrillation and get Purser the ablation treatment he needed. Months after his procedure, the Houston man was back at his workout routine—including virtual boxing.

Compared to wearing a Holter or event monitor for weeks to a month, wearing a smartwatch is relatively nonintrusive, comfortable, and less expensive. One added benefit of having a portable ECG with you at nearly all times? Getting the data that would be necessary to jump-start the medical process to confirm a diagnosis. For disorders like atrial fibrillation where an earlier diagnosis can mean the difference between a curative therapy and permanent heart damage, that time savings can be priceless.

A View from Center Court

For nearly my entire career, my job has been to peer down the pike and tell my employer, fellow executives, or investors which products or business model will be the next best thing in healthcare. In my thirty years in life sciences and healthcare, I've helped companies produce technologies that have impacted the health of hundreds of thousands of patients. I've advised corporations like Sony and Samsung on how to bring their technology into the medical space, and I've helped multinationals like GE identify and develop new, emerging businesses in healthcare and life sciences.

Today, I am a general partner at a venture capital firm, where we find and fund promising tech companies that use AI and big data to make diagnostic devices, new therapies, and other high-impact products. This means I'm constantly reviewing the next wave of technologies that could disrupt healthcare, putting me in the unique position to judge what's coming next—which is what you'll find, in part, detailed throughout this book.

Today, every major tech company worth its digital salt is trying to find a way to grow its data and get or expand into the healthcare space. Healthcare spending currently accounts for 17.7 percent of the US's Gross Domestic Product (GDP), and these tech companies all want a piece of the pie. Here's how several of the world's top tech giants are making a play into forecasting your future health:

> Apple: Apple has been heavily involved in AI-driven healthcare since 2014, when it launched its Health app, which now comes preinstalled on all iPhones. Today, Apple has a bevy of products designed to help you take better control of your health, whenever and wherever you want. Not only can Apple Watch take an ECG, it can also alert doctors if you fall, tell you when you're most fertile, read your blood oxygen (O_2) levels, and donate all your personal data (with your permission, of course) to science in the name of medical research. On the horizon? Apple is rumored to be adding blood glucose reading to the Watch. Imagine the ability to monitor your blood sugar levels

accurately just by wearing your watch, without having to prick your fingers every few hours. Apple is also designing devices for doctors, including those that allow physicians to monitor sick patients at home. Here's what Apple CEO Tim Cook told CNBC's Jim Cramer in 2019: "I believe, if you zoom out into the future and you look back and you ask the question, 'What was Apple's greatest contribution to mankind?', it will be about health."

Google: No name is more synonymous with high tech than Google and its parent company, Alphabet. Its healthcare ambitions don't always spring to mind, but the conglomerate is also behind Verily Life Sciences (Alphabet's life sciences research arm and developer of the Verily Study Watch, a smartwatch designed for clinical trial patient monitoring) and DeepMind (the AI subsidiary that created AlphaFold, which predicts protein structures). At the 2020 World Economic Forum in Davos, Switzerland, Alphabet CEO Sundar Pichai told a conference panel that healthcare has the biggest potential to improve patient outcomes over the next five to ten years using AI. While Pichai recognizes that the data needed to improve patient outcomes rests in the hands of the hospitals, he gets it. "Look at the potential here," he told the panel. "Cancer is often missed, and the difference in outcome is profound. In lung cancer, for example, five experts agree this way and five agree the other way. We know we can use artificial intelligence to make it better."

Amazon: Over the last few years, Amazon has been quietly toiling away at an app that could sell you medical services like doctor's appointments, virtual telehealth visits, and pharmaceuticals as easily as the online retailer pedals you books, baby strollers, and whatever else you could possibly want. And the tech behemoth recently launched its Amazon Halo health band, a screenless health and fitness (and more) tracker. Why would you trust former Amazon CEO Jeff Bezos with your life, as *Newsweek* rightfully asked in a 2019 cover story, "Dr. Amazon?" Right now, Amazon lets you shop for the best products at the best price from the comfort of your couch. Imagine if you could do the same for your healthcare, with complete price transparency—something that doesn't exist in today's medical world. A senior healthcare industry analyst at the research firm Forrester told Newsweek: "Healthcare has never been a shoppable industry. Amazon is going to change that."

Facebook: In 2016, Facebook CEO Mark Zuckerberg announced he and his wife were committing a whopping $3 billion to cure every disease by the end of the century. Since then, the tech mogul has stealthily been making his foray into healthcare. Facebook, with two-billion-plus users worldwide, already uses AI to mine user posts for indicators of mental-health problem like depression and suicidal tendencies. The social media conglomerate also recently launched a healthcare platform to help users keep track of their doctor appointments and send checkup reminders for preventive screenings. Facebook has also partnered with research teams to develop new data-driven products, including an AI-enabled machine that will decrease how long it takes to get an MRI. Late to enter the wearable race, Facebook is said to be working on a new smartwatch that would launch sometime in 2022 and would give users messaging alongside the standard fitness capabilities.

Microsoft: Not to be outdone by the other tech giants in its cyber sandbox, Microsoft is also accelerating into data-driven healthcare. In 2020, the software titan launched "AI for Health," a $40-million program to help hospitals and other healthcare providers improve patient care using AI and big data. To that end, Microsoft already has 169,000 contracts with different healthcare organizations around the world. The company, like other tech conglomerates, sees its entrée into healthcare as altruistic, democratizing medicine with its digital reach. According to Dr. Peter Lee, corporate vice president of Microsoft Healthcare: "Four billion people on this planet today have no reasonable access to healthcare. AI and technology have to be part of the solution to creating that more equitable access."

NVIDIA: You might not think that a gaming tech company would have a lot to do with healthcare, but you'd be mistaken. NVIDIA, perhaps best known for developing graphics processing units (GPUs) that make video games seem realistic, is using its computing platforms to help doctors better detect disease, screen drug compounds, and improve medical imaging interpretation. In fact, its healthcare and life sciences division is working on solutions that address many of the problems I'll describe in later chapters, from building smart hospitals to developing precision medicine based on genomics.

The Fine Print Below the Promise

We all have the chance to let AI and big data make us healthier and happier in some way. But beneath every promise is always a little bit of fine print, and all this technology won't come free of cost for humanity. There will be a social and economic toll. And issues like data privacy and the ethical consequences of AI-enabled healthcare will keep these topics in the public discourse for some time to come.

As much as data-driven technology will overhaul patient outcomes, it will also upend the current economics and culture of medicine. Quite frankly, the entire life sciences industry will be turned upside down and inside out as AI changes how we, the public, interact with the healthcare system, expect drug and vaccine discovery to happen on a much shorter timeframe, and demand healthcare costs decrease. Hospitals, doctors, drug manufacturers, and insurance companies will be forced to adapt or retire from practice. Medical training will need to adapt, and medical school might look more like math class than today's traditional training. Where today's medical students get training on how to navigate electronic health records, tomorrow's students will learn how to use AI and analytics to identify at-risk patient populations, prescribe the best medication for a patient, or practice an operation dozens of times, virtually encountering potential complications, long before meeting the patient on the operating table. Some people will have to be reschooled. Others who cannot adapt will lose their jobs.

Like any revolution, there will also be Luddites, or those who resist change. Many will be mistrustful of data-driven devices and refuse to use the new technology. When speaking about how AI and big data will disrupt healthcare, I've already been accused of heresy by several irate physicians. I get it: there's a lot of fear, and many wonder whether doctors will still be relevant in the age of AI (hint: they will be).

To this end, providers and patients alike will face new challenges over the significance of human interaction and how to negotiate the value difference between man and machine. Ethical questions, especially surrounding genetics, will also arise. For example, if you can edit a gene that causes a disease in a fetus, why not edit others for hair color, creativity, or propensity toward athletic performance?

These are just a smattering of the considerations we'll all face in the age of AI, with some of us already facing them. What to do? Knowledge is power, and while I didn't say it:

> *"Educating yourself is the passport to the future, for tomorrow belongs to those who prepare for it today."—Malcolm X, human rights activist*

As a patient and healthcare consumer, you can either avoid or ignore the dramatic changes that are happening—or you can learn everything you can about what's happening to healthcare so that you know how to navigate it and can take advantage of what the new technology has to offer.

Remember when you got your first smartphone and texting seemed weird? Or when FaceTime and Google Hangouts became commonplace? Well, imagine if you never learned how to text or use video chat. That's what ignoring technology and AI in your quest to be healthier would be like. These things are already happening, and you can choose to ignore them or use them to your advantage. If you understand how these different technologies can help you, you can help yourself, your family, and your friends to live healthier. It's not just about maximizing our lifespan, it's about increasing our healthspan. So, it's time to video-call your doctor and type out a text to yourself:

This is how you take charge of your future well-being. ☺
This is the path to *The Future You.*

CHAPTER ONE:

ON THE BRINK OF A MEDICAL REVOLUTION

"Artificial intelligence is one of the most profound things we're working on as humanity. It is more profound than fire or electricity."
—Sundar Pichai, CEO of Alphabet Inc (Google)

Artificial intelligence is transforming every aspect of our society—and at an incredible rate. This includes which kind of jobs we work, how we manage our money, how we teach our children, what kind of cars we drive (or don't drive), how we interact with our families and friends, how we shop, and how we spend our precious leisure time.

More and more CEOs are seeing the power of AI. Banks know the power of AI. The US government is slowly learning the power of AI, and so is the media, with *The New York Times, The Wall Street Journal, Fortune,* and other eminent publications all issuing special reports on AI in the past six months alone. The technology's importance was also underscored by the coronavirus outbreak, when AI became critical to developing statistical models and manufacturing a vaccine. Healthcare today is relying on AI to keep us healthier and treat us faster. And whether we realize it or not, we also know the power of AI when our Grubhub recommendation for pad thai hits the spot, or when we discover a new favorite author or clothing brand.

But what exactly is AI? According to a recent Gallup poll, 85 percent of Americans use the technology regularly, even though many don't realize it or have any idea what it is.

This chapter will try to demystify the basics of AI technology and show you how it's already part of our everyday lives, with real-world examples. For example, the navigation app you use every day on your phone to help you avoid traffic? Enabled by AI. The smart thermostat you use to control your home's environment from your phone? Powered by AI. The smart kitchen you see in futuristic films, complete with a self-restocking refrigerator, windows that give a digitized view of whatever you want, and a robot that cleans, cooks, and serves you? You start to see the significance. Pretty soon, it won't be a stretch to say that our daily lives are brought to us by AI.

Here, we'll explore the different subsets of AI, including machine learning and deep learning. We'll define big data, with real-world examples of both structured (something that fits in a nice, neat box) and unstructured (think of this as something freeform that can't be easily standardized) data and provide a brief history of exactly how information became so massive—and valuable. We'll also outline how AI and big data are now coming together in a perfect storm to bring us to where we are now—on the brink of a major medical revolution.

In addition to an upheaval in healthcare, AI and big data are also causing the world's fourth industrial revolution, an idea corroborated by economists. Together, AI and big data will change our lives, whether we embrace the technology or not. Here, we'll look at how AI and big data will transform us financially, socially, and culturally, upending even the basic ideology of what it means to be human.

The Periodic Table of AI

It can sometimes seem that doctors speak a completely foreign language than the rest of us. Have you ever been in an elevator and overheard a conversation between two doctors or researchers? They could be speaking in Martian, for all I know. That's even more apparent if you ask an expert in biotech or a computer scientist to explain what they do. If only there was a Google Translate setting for "science or technical or medical" to "regular person"!

That disconnect in the language that scientists and doctors use and how the rest of us talk has some negative consequences. For one thing, some of the discoveries and advances are utterly mind-blowing and deserve front-page newspaper positions or at least have a tweet about it go viral—if you can break through the science-speak. In this book, I'm going to try to translate some of the technical jargon into something that makes more sense to the rest of us.

Let's start with AI. What it is, what it isn't, and how many different ways we can talk about it.

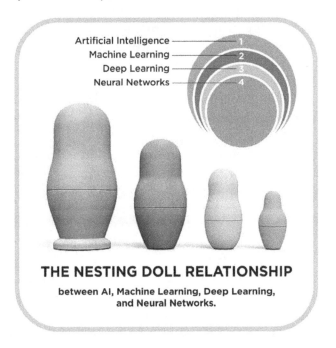

Figure 1.1. The nesting doll relationship between AI, machine learning, deep learning, and neural networks.

There are probably as many definitions of AI as there are scientists who work on it. But in general, AI is a variety of techniques for getting computers to process information similarly to the way a human might. The different methods are a bit like Russian matryoshka, or nesting dolls. For example, machine learning is a subset of AI that uses methods to get a computer to "learn" on its own, and deep learning is a specific kind of machine learning.

Neural networks make up the majority of deep-learning algorithms—they attempt to mimic how the human brain works. For every decision you make (or really, anything you do), the neurons in your brain fire. Some neural pathways are short, and others are long and complex, causing multiple neurons to fire in a precise sequence. If you turn your head to the left, different neurons will fire than if you turn it to the right. This is the idea behind artificial neural networks: for every piece of data, the input that the network is fed, the computer can get to an answer, the output (Figure 1.2).

What do the input and outputs look like? How do scientists actually do AI?

Math.

Scientists use algorithms to work in AI (and more specifically, machine learning, deep learning, and neural networks). An algorithm is like a sentence made of mathematical symbols or numbers instead of words:

$$\sum_{i=1}^{n} a_i x_i + \beta = P$$

If you ever took advanced algebra or calculus in school, those symbols might look vaguely familiar. Fortunately for you and me, we don't have to get into the details of the math—it's enough to understand that when I write about a machine learning algorithm, you can imagine that a series of mathematical sentences is behind it. The concepts behind the algorithms can be fairly simple (is this a picture of an apple?) to more complicated (what's the likelihood I'll go see a movie tonight?). But no matter how complex the question is, you can be sure that there's a lot of math and computer science getting to the answer.

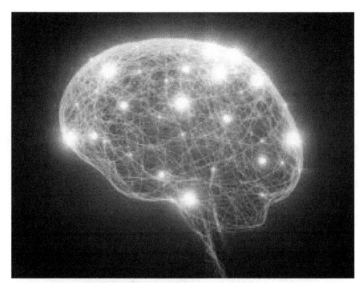

Structure of a neural network

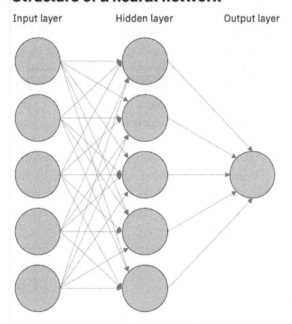

Figure 1.2. The complexity of artificial neural networks (right) and similarity to neural networks in the brain (left). [top image source: IBM; bottom image source: Google]

If those definitions seem a little vague, or you're still not quite sure what they mean, raise your hand. Hand in the air? You're not alone. What might be easier is to describe AI by all the things it is used for and can do. And keep in mind that what follows are just examples of what AI can do today. In the future? The sky's the limit.

In 2016, IBM joined forces with the XPRIZE Foundation to launch a challenge to use AI for the greater good. The competition, which is scheduled to announce the grand prize winner(s) in 2021, was designed to use AI to improve human life. From a starting field of one hundred and fifty international teams, ten semifinalists are using AI in a variety of ways: creating an application for doctors and patients to tackle mental health (Aifred Health, Canada); robots that sort recyclables (CleanRobotics, US); building an AI-enabled pancreas for patients with unstable Type 1 diabetes (Team MachineGenes, Australia); and using facial and pattern recognition to find missing children and stop sex trafficking (Traffic Jam by Marinus Analytics, US). You can already see that AI is being used for a wide variety of applications that go far beyond healthcare. It's not hyperbole when I say that AI truly is or will soon be able to affect nearly every aspect of your life—whether you know it or not.

In 2017, Dr. Kristian Hammond, a professor of computer science at Northwestern University, published the "Periodic Table of AI" for the IBM Watson XPRIZE AI competition's web page. Hammond's conception looks a lot like a shortened version of the periodic table of elements that you may remember from high school chemistry. As you move from left to right and top to bottom across the figure, the complexity of the task increases.

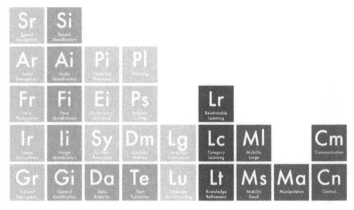

Figure 1.3. The Periodic Table of AI by Dr. Kris Hammond.

Imagine that you buy a house, and in the attic you find a very old audio tape and player. When you press play, as a human you can generally tell if the sounds coming from the machine are someone talking (even if it's in another language), music playing, or random noise. AI can do this too. These are the items on the far top left of the Periodic Table of AI: speech and audio recognition. If you move to the right, you have speech identification. To go back to our old tape example, that would be like figuring out that the tape is a conversation in English or Russian, or that it's a piano versus a violin. When you ask Alexa or Siri to find out the name and artist of a song you're listening to, you're using AI for audio identification. It's not just recognizing that there's something to listen to—Siri can tell you if Taylor Swift or the Beatles are playing.

Facial recognition is still more complex than speech or audio recognition, but recognizing something like a face is still less complicated than both image recognition (one step down) or facial identification (one step to the right). Even though speech recognition and identification are at the top on the left, you can see that actually understanding the conversation on that tape is a much more complex task for a computer to do—even though you probably don't think anything of it for your native language.

At the bottom far right is control. Remember HAL 9000, the AI computer that takes control of the spaceship from the movie *2001: A Space Odyssey*? This is probably what most of us think of when we joke about our "AI overlords." But you can see there are a lot of ways that AI can be used in between speech recognition and an AI system becoming sentient (and bent on controlling humanity).

In this chapter and throughout the book, you'll see that sometimes I'll describe something as AI and sometimes as machine learning or deep learning or neural network or some other term in the AI toolbox. Where a specific technique is used, like machine learning to predict if a patient will develop a condition or a neural network to analyze medical imaging to find tiny cancers, I'll use the word that is specific. And when multiple methods are being used for a particular task, or if it's not clear, I'll use the more general "AI." No matter what the term is, it's all AI.

Your Perfect Personal Shopper

Have you ever spent a night out with friends and the next day, your Facebook or Instagram feed is full of ads for exactly the things you talked about? You'd be in good company if you have felt a little creeped out by how perfectly your social media ads target you. Is your phone spying on you? Is Facebook listening in on your conversations?

Chances are, probably not. What is happening is that advertisers are using AI to target consumers at a microlevel. While some companies will still use general demographic information (males ages thirty to forty-five living in Chicago) and blanket everyone who meets that basic criteria, other companies are looking to increase their odds of getting a new customer with hyperfocused information that can feel like you're being spied on. How are they doing this? It all comes down to AI and big data.

What is "big data" exactly? Imagine the biggest, most complex spreadsheet you've ever thought of. Every piece of information about you (and everyone else) would be in that spreadsheet—from when and where you were born, to how long you've lived in your current house, to whether or not you buy store brands at the grocery store. A lot of the data is what we'd call structured—it's information that has a consistent format. Telephone numbers, Social Security numbers, even dates, are structured data.

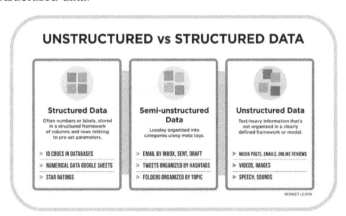

Figure 1.4. Structured vs. unstructured data examples.
[Adapted from: https://monkeylearn.com/blog/structured-data-vs-unstructured-data/]

Computers are really good at crunching through structured data, but not all information can be easily categorized or put into a structured format. Information that doesn't fit neatly into the structured data box is (not surprisingly) unstructured. Examples of unstructured data might include the names of all of the books you read last year, your favorite song, or your favorite vacation place. Sometimes there are ways of turning unstructured data into something that is structured. That list of books? Instead of titles, they could be listed as ISBN codes (those numbers and bar codes on the backs of books). Your favorite beach? Turned into a GPS location.

Big data is used to help AI do the kinds of tasks that the Periodic Table of AI lists, while AI makes sense of big data. The two go hand in hand. The bigger and richer the data set (remember: think gigantic spreadsheet), the better the AI can be at doing its thing.

Whether we realize it or not, pretty much everything we do leaves a data trail, and that information is what companies are using to reach us. Girls night out at a local wine bar? You could be leaving data crumbs that suggest you're more likely to drink wine than beer. Combined with other information, like GPS location information, shopping habits and history, your information, and that of millions of other people, AI starts to paint a pretty good picture of someone who is fifty-three years old, lives in Manhattan, buys premium dog food but store brands for groceries, splurges once a year on a trip someplace tropical, and probably would enjoy learning about a new app that helps people pair their dinners or chocolate with wine suggestions. As unique as we all are, in advertisers' eyes, we're just another data point.

I don't want to give you the impression that it's a piece of cake to combine all of that information. It's not— today. Your grocery store might have your food shopping history because you signed up for coupons and its frequent shopper program to get discounts, but it probably isn't sharing that information (either anonymously or aggregated with other shoppers' data) with companies. However, some of our behaviors around social media make it easier to do this. We willingly post about seeing a particular movie, eating certain types of food at particular restaurants, or traveling to specific vacation destinations. It's not so hard, then, for advertisers to send us the hypertargeted ads that make us wonder if someone is spying on us. I'll come back to some of these ideas later in Chapter Nine.

Feeding the Planet

What do you think of when you hear the word "farmer"? Someone with a few acres and a garden with dozens of different vegetables and maybe a few fruit trees? Agriculture looks a lot different than it did a century ago, when the small-scale farmer was the standard. Today, farmers are challenged to produce enough food for the almost eight billion of us on the planet in the face of climate change and development. And they're doing it with AI.

Just like we humans produce data, farms do too. Want to know the best place to plant wheat? Analyze a few years' worth of information about rainfall, sunlight, and soil to figure out the best wheat strain to plant. Need a tomato that can be picked early so that by the time it gets to market, it's perfectly ripe? You need data and maybe some genetic engineering—made possible by AI. Want to figure out the best crop rotation schedule? AI can help you with that.

Today's farms are just as likely to hire a data scientist as they are someone to pick the fruit—especially if they want to be successful. Fields are mapped by GPS, drones take pictures to monitor insect or animal damage, and rainfall is measured by wireless- and Bluetooth-connected devices. Insecticides and pesticides can be targeted to specific rows or even individual plants. Fertilizer use can be reduced, because it doesn't need to be spread across an entire field—maybe only a section or two. Workers can be hired to pick the produce at exactly the right time to bring it to market, and their labor can be scheduled to move from farm to farm more efficiently.

It's not just large corporate farms that are taking advantage of AI and big data. Small farmers might be in even more need to maximize their yields and protect their crops from insects, birds, inclement weather, or seemingly unexplained failure. This is the idea behind the ag-tech start-up IntelinAir. The company has developed a platform it calls AGMRI to help farmers maximize crop yields. Similar to how radiologists look at MRI images to diagnose illness, the AGMRI platform uses images collected by drones that fly over fields more than a dozen times per year. These high-resolution images are combined with data from a variety of sources, from topographic maps to weather forecasts to soil analysis, using deep learning algorithms. The result? A system that can sense when parts of a crop are under stress—while there is still time to intervene with things like extra watering and nutrients, or which parts of a field might need some weeding or targeted pesticide application. By collecting this data over time, year after year, farmers can better identify which crops might grow best in certain locations, which fertilizers or pesticides work best with the least negative impact, and when to plant and harvest at precise times.

Where Are You Going?

One of the most exciting ideas in global planning is the idea of smart cities. Imagine heading to New York City or Los Angeles and never being stuck in traffic; cities where pedestrians, cyclists, cars, and public transportation work together seamlessly to get people from Point A to Point B more efficiently. Where vehicle crashes are a thing of the past. By now, you've probably guessed that AI has something to do with making that vision a reality.

The technology company NVIDIA and researchers at leading universities around the world have organized the AI City Challenge since 2017. The competition's aims change each year and are focused on using AI to solve some of the headaches of city planners and departments of transportation. How to correctly estimate the speed of traffic, classify what types of vehicles use the road, and how to identify pedestrians and predict their behavior at intersections are just a few of its challenge goals.

Results over the five years of AI City Challenges are things that are already in play—in some locations, at a basic non-AI level. Ever sit at a red light when there's no traffic in any direction in the middle of the night? It would be great to have lights that could detect the fact that it's 3 a.m., and you're the only vehicle on the street in a two-mile radius, so the lights automatically sync to green as you approach each intersection. Some cities already take the time of day into consideration for traffic light timing, leaving one direction green for a long time, while the cross streets have the long red. Others have sensors at the top of the streetlights that use approaching vehicle headlights to keep a green light green or turn a red light to green.

Sensors and timers aren't AI, but they can be used with AI to make traffic safer. For example, that 3 a.m. car that's the only vehicle on the road for miles? It might still get a red light if the traffic cameras pick up a pedestrian or cyclist that will be crossing the street at the same time. Get the car to stop, and the chances of an accident go down. That would require more complexity than simply identifying that there's a pedestrian walking at a steady pace who will reach the intersection in four minutes, precisely when the vehicle will get there, because the AI system would have to "know" this and also predict that the driver won't stop in time, so it will turn the light red early enough that the driver wouldn't try to speed through the intersection on a yellow (or even turn the light red at the intersection before this one).

CityFlow is the name given to the data set used in the AI City Challenges. What does the data look like? It's the aggregation of video captured by forty cameras from ten intersections in a medium-sized US city over three hours. In addition to the actual video, the data set also includes annotations (Figure).

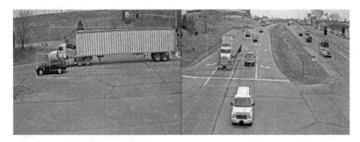

Figure 1.5. Image from CityFlow data set, with red lines showing the relationship between objects from different perspectives. [Tang et al.]

Above, you can see that the two pictures are of the same SUV and tractor trailer, shown from cameras with different perspectives. Teaching an AI system to recognize that these are the same vehicles is powerful. It's similar to the training we all help with when we are asked to type in Captcha codes or pick the boxes that contain numbers, letters, or some object. It's also a lot like how toddlers learn that both cats and dogs are animals, but cats are cats, dogs are dogs, and tigers are cats, not dogs. That kind of discrimination might seem pretty obvious and simple to an adult, but training a computer to do it correctly all of the time, with billions of objects, is an incredible undertaking.

Now think about a busy intersection in your town—two lanes of traffic moving in each direction with a dedicated right turn lane for each street. Imagine you and three of your friends were to each stand at a different corner of the intersection and watch the traffic go by for five minutes. At the end of that time, a blue truck runs a red light, narrowly missing a brown car moving across the intersection, and continues down the road. How would each of you describe that scene to a police officer? You'd have four different perspectives and ways of telling the same story.

One of the AI City Challenges is to help AI understand that each of those perspectives and descriptions are telling one true version of the same story. Natural language processing, or language understanding (see the Periodic Table of AI, above), is something we've only recently gotten good at training computers to do. One of the best examples is when IBM Watson won the *Jeopardy!* game show. The computer system had to be able to understand, or process, the questions posed by the late host Alex Trebek.

In a recent paper, three researchers from Boston University and the University of Washington explain what that looks like for the AI City Challenge. For each vehicle, the researchers have created three descriptions. For example, using the figure above, descriptions might be "A black SUV is sitting at a traffic light,"; "The dark SUV is next to the tractor trailer"; and, "The gray SUV overtakes the semi in the intersection." Depending on your vantage point and the exact moment in time you look, each of those statements might be true (or at least true from your perspective).

In simple terms, training an AI system might go something like this. Let's say you want to be able to have the AI correctly identify specific car models and estimate their model year (Image Identification, in the Periodic Table of AI). You could imagine law enforcement agencies might find an AI application that could do this pretty useful for bank robberies or Amber Alerts. You might start by training the AI with images from car manufacturers. For each image you have, you would tell the computer, "This is a 2017 Nissan Rogue"; or "This isn't a 2017 Nissan Rogue/This is a 2014 Volvo XC40." Pictures of the vehicles in different colors, trim packages, and from different angles would be useful.

In the end, you wouldn't need an example of every single option for every year a vehicle was made. Why not? Because you would train the AI to learn on its own (Category Learning). Give it enough examples of different cars (a training set), and then let it categorize the rest on its own (a testing set). Humans "fact-check" what the AI gives back. Maybe it does a great job at differentiating between cars and SUVs but mixes up the SUV models too often if it only sees the back end of the vehicle from an angle. A new training round, focusing on SUVs, viewed from that position, could put the AI back on track. The real test comes when you turn the AI system on to a data set that it hasn't seen before, like CityFlow, any number of the ones used for training autonomous vehicles, or even real-world data.

In fact, autonomous, or self-driving, vehicles present one of the biggest applications of AI and highlight the difficulties engineers are facing. Imagine you're driving down your neighborhood street on the way downtown. When you see a speed limit or traffic sign, you know how fast you should be going and what to do at the intersection. Automotive manufacturers can put sensors and cameras on cars that pick up on those signs—remember the AI Periodic Table? The AI would use image recognition (That is a stop sign. This is a traffic light.) alongside some programmed rules (Stop the vehicle at the stop sign. Continue through the intersection if the traffic light is green.) that tell the car what to do. Given the right training, you could imagine programming the car to travel to a destination and then just sitting back and enjoying the ride.

What becomes more difficult is teaching the AI system how to interpret competing inputs and managing certain situations, like a crash that can't be avoided without someone being hurt. Every other driver on the road, every person near an intersection, or even road debris and potholes add to the number of inputs—and therefore the complexity—of the algorithms needed to train the AI system.

This description of how to train the AI isn't specific to cars and trucks. The basic format (train, test, repeat) is roughly the same for everything from speech recognition and image identification to understanding language and the foundation for things like chatbots and apps that determine whether or not you have a genetic disorder from a picture of your face.

Our Jetsons Moment

Growing up watching *The Jetsons*, I always wondered when things like flying cars, robot housekeepers, and kitchens that delivered entire meals at the push of a button would go from sci-fi cartoons to real life. While flying cars may still be some time to come, we're edging closer with self-driving cars, and we already have robot vacuums and meal delivery services like Grubhub feeding us at the click of our mouse. AI is the backbone to all of this. Our Jetsons moment may not be far off.

AI is bringing us toward what I (and others) am calling the Fourth Industrial Revolution. What do I mean by that? It's the combination of AI with other technologies, like 3D printing and the Internet of Things, to automate manufacturing and industry. Klaus Schwab, head of the World Economic Forum, coined the phrase and wrote a book on the topic.

Like the three industrial revolutions that came before, this revolution is marked by a relatively rapid gain of technologies that utterly transform how life was before. The first industrial revolution brought about the use of steam and waterpower to shift manufacturing from entirely human-driven to machines, while the second brought about the expansion of electricity and telegraph cables across the country and around the world. The latest industrial revolution occurred more recently, at the end of the twentieth century, and is sometimes referred to as the Digital Revolution, due to its emphasis on digitizing data and adoption of computers.

The Fourth Industrial Revolution is catapulting us forward in ways we can't even imagine. Every aspect of our lives will be irrevocably altered.

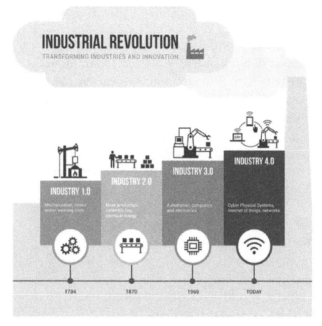

Figure 1.6. Evolution of the Industrial Revolutions.
[https://spacenews.com/sponsored/industrial-revolution/]

The Future You: TikTok, AI, and You

After several decades, it's clear that computers and all the technology that came afterward have made our lives both better and worse in different ways. We've gained literally years of productivity and efficiency while complaining how teenagers' eyes are glued to their phones and no one wants to have a phone conversation anymore. Sharing information happens in thirty-second TikTok videos that go viral, while local newspapers are shutting down the presses. New job roles and entirely new industries have sprung up as some workers are made redundant.

Today, we're on the cusp of a new era driven by technology that is truly science fiction brought to life. The Fourth Industrial Revolution. Every aspect of life is transforming—from how we shop, travel, and bank, to how we feed the nearly eight billion people on this planet—and it's being reshaped in ways that we are only now beginning to comprehend.

One of the most exciting areas of new research ponders the fundamental philosophical question, "What does it mean to be human?" We might think we know the answer to this—maybe something about our emotions, our awareness of self and others, or our insatiable curiosity and desire to push boundaries. But when we combine AI technology, engineering, and the human body, those lines that define Man vs. Machine break down.

Poor eyesight? We have implantable lenses, corneas, or retinas that correct vision and can work like built-in telescopes. Trouble hearing your partner over the TV? How about hearing aids that never need a new battery, are completely hidden, and adjust automatically—or even undergo a new gene therapy technique to restore your hearing? Loss of a hand, foot, or entire arm or leg? Why not have a prosthetic one, 3D printed, that literally feels like your own skin, provides the same sensations, and that you can control without thinking. Feeling great? Wouldn't it be fantastic to have a built-in check-engine light to warn you that your blood sugar is too high or you're in the early stages of coronary artery disease—and what you can do to reverse it? It's the Six Million Dollar Man or Inspector Gadget brought to life—made possible because of AI.

Think it's all too far-fetched? True, some of these things aren't quite ready for prime time or past early stages of development. But work that originally started to support combat veterans with amputations has pushed prosthetic research beyond what was possible even a few years ago, and others are closer to reality than you might imagine. We even see Olympians running with prosthetic legs.

Are You Ready for the Future?

The ways in which AI is reshaping the health and wellness industries are earth-shattering, and I want everyone to see what I do every day, as I work to find promising start-ups and ideas in this space. Everyone has a vested interest in staying healthy—and what I'm going to share in the following chapters matters to *you*. Whether you're trying to finally lose those stubborn ten pounds for good, want to understand why your cholesterol medication is causing you to have leg pains, help you navigate a new diagnosis, or just want to learn something, *The Future You* is your guidebook to what comes next.

I hope that this chapter has given you some concrete examples of how AI is already transforming our world, even if we don't realize it. The food we eat, the cars we drive, the things we buy—AI is helping farmers get more food out of their harvests, making our roads safer, and giving us more of the products we really want.

In the upcoming chapters, I'll describe how AI isn't only a part of some futuristic vision of our world—I'll show you how you can take advantage of the things AI is doing to improve your life now. AI is giving you a gentle nudge when you need to eat a little healthier or remind you that it's time for a checkup. AI is your personal coach, encouraging you through a tough workout or suggesting how to improve your yoga form. When you get sick, AI is helping you find the best doctor that takes your insurance and has an opening this afternoon or telling you that your problem is serious enough to warrant a trip to an urgent care or emergency room. AI is discovering new medications and making sure the right patient gets it at the right time. Think of AI as your own personal shopper and wellness coach in one. Let's get started.

CHAPTER TWO:

HOW DATA CAN MAKE YOU FITTER, LEANER, AND LESS STRESSED

"Health is a state of body. Wellness is a state of being."—J. *Stanford, author*

Raise your hand if you'd like to lose a few pounds, get better sleep, or just more generally be healthier. If you asked this question in a room filled with people, nearly everyone would have their hand up. After all, who doesn't this apply to? The idea that tools like AI can learn to help you eat better, get fit, lose weight, sleep more, lower stress, and be happier as a result is perhaps the one of the sexiest sells the technology has today, as millions look to optimize their wellness. Today, wellness is a $4 trillion industry, with Americans spending more money on gym memberships and diet plans than they do on college tuition. Tech companies want a piece of the pie and already have plenty of products to offer.

Countless AI-enabled smartphone apps and sensors already exist in the wellness space, which helped colonize the world of wearables with Fitbit and other step counters. Not only can you track your steps today, you can also map your runs, hikes, bikes, and swims using AI-enabled apps, which will coach you through everything from boxing classes and weight workouts to surf lessons and many different forms of meditation. If you want to eat better, apps will track your calories, plan your meals, and answer all your questions via a chatbot nutritionist. If you want to lose weight, apps will help pick the best meals and suggest exercise routines; monitor your blood sugar, body fat, and other biometrics; and provide coaching whenever you need it. Apps that monitor sleep are already popular, and you'll find hundreds of apps and sensors that work to lower stress and even change brain-wave activity.

This is what AI can do now. In the future, AI-enabled software will tailor-fit your nutrition, exercise, sleep, and stress to your personal data, including your genomics, environment, lifestyle, and even molecular biology, like the health of your microbiome. This will allow computers to craft specific recommendations for you, like whether a keto diet or calorie-controlled plan will help you lose weight, or if you should do a strength or cardio workout for optimal fitness.

In this chapter, I'll show you just how far AI and machine learning have come in the health and wellness space: Devices like smart mirrors that coach you through workouts while monitoring your biometrics in order to give you a more effective sweat session. Virtual-reality headsets or gyms that let you catch a pass from Tom Brady or take a yoga class on a beach in Bali. AI-designed meals, tailored to the specific macro- and micronutrients you need to stay healthy or lose weight, and that are shipped to your door. Apps that integrate scientifically proven methods to help you relax, improve depression, and get you to sleep. The future isn't far off—it's already here.

Map My Sport: How AI and Apps Have Transformed Exercise into a Group Challenge

It's no secret that group activities are beneficial for health and wellness. But after high school or college, few among us continue to play team sports, as life gets in the way and our exercise pursuits become more solitary. Tech companies know this and have designed apps and products to bring us back to the fun, competitive nature of team play.

In boutique gyms like Orangetheory and SoulCycle, your workout comes with the added boost of leader boards, showing you exactly where you rank among your fellow athletes. While achieving personal goals, folks who are motivated by some friendly competition (if not the good-natured trash talk of the courts) will find incentive to pedal faster or run harder to reach the top. But not everyone can or wants to work out at a gym. Thankfully, you don't have to give up your competitive nature if you cancel your gym membership.

In the face of the COVID-19 pandemic, when gyms across the country closed for weeks and months at a time, exercise tech companies saw demand for their products soar as people contemplated the effects of shelter-in-place restrictions. Peloton Interactive, manufacturer of exercise bikes and treadmills and an interactive app, is one example. The pricey equipment comes with large screens for users to follow along as upbeat coaches direct their workouts, which end with a class ranking. Prefer to focus on individual achievements instead of competition? You'll be awarded badges for consistency and frequency of working out.

You don't need expensive equipment to reap the benefits of exercise competition, however. Running and cycling may be among the best examples of how to make even low-tech methods competitive and entertaining, with apps like MapMyRun, Strava, and CityStrides. Though these sports are well known for high-profile races, such as the Boston Marathon or Tour de France, professional athletes and weekend warriors alike are using these apps and others to challenge fellow users to run or bike a certain number of miles per month, scale an equivalent height to Mount Everest, or achieve a personal best time over a set distance.

Strava, MapMyRun, Fitbit, Garmin, and dozens of other apps collect workout data from wearable devices and match it to your GPS location, drawing a map of your route, from hiking in the woods to running the streets of San Francisco or Madrid. Many of them let you share your workout information with others on their platforms, something like an early Facebook wall—but focused only on workout activities. Want to brag about running the London Marathon at an astonishingly fast pace or let friends and family track your progress as you hike the

Appalachian Trail? These apps let you do exactly that. In some groups, if it isn't documented on Strava, it might as well have not even happened. Want to show off your creative side? Strava users can design workouts that look like dinosaurs, teddy bears, or even a marriage proposal (Figure 2.1), and some of the attempts have garnered attention from the media.

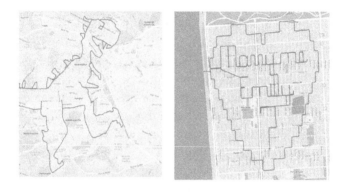

Figure 2.1. Strava Art submitted by Strava users to stravart website [https://www.strav.art]

Whether you want the camaraderie of group fitness, a way to replicate the gym experience at home, or a platform for documenting your personal best in solo pursuits, these websites and apps (along with a variety of wearable GPS trackers and smartphones) can help you achieve your goals.

Sidebar:
How Strava Sent the US Military into a Panic

San Francisco-based Strava estimated that it has twenty-seven million unique users worldwide, each leaving behind their GPS trail of activities. Every few months, Strava releases a "heatmap" of aggregated routes of publicly available workouts. Map areas with more activity show up as brighter in intensity, while areas that have little to none will be dark (Figure 2.2). The data is a visually stunning snapshot of workouts around the world, and data geeks can drill down to street-level detail. You might be able to figure out where the local high schools are by finding the very bright, tiny perfect ovals, even if you didn't use the street names to guide you, and you can trace the Chicago or Berlin Marathon routes, run by tens of thousands, and not just on the days of the races.

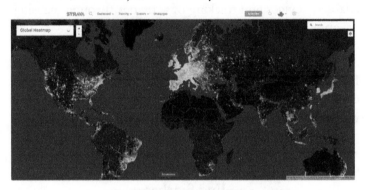

Figure 2.2. Strava heatmap of activities.
[https://www.strava.com/heatmap#7.00/-120.90000/38.36000/hot/all]

Although the heatmap is pretty neat from a data visualization standpoint, with over a billion running and cycling activities encompassing thirteen trillion GPS points, it's not difficult to see that some users might have a problem with adding their data to the mix and opt to keep their workout information private. Finding the local high school is interesting, but not likely to be a national security threat. It's this latter issue that Strava realized in early 2018, when the late 2017 version of its heatmap faced scrutiny.

You can imagine the concern, then, when people started to realize that secret military bases and intelligence locations might be discovered by finding areas of activity in places that should have otherwise been dark.

An Australian National University student, Nathan Ruser, set off a flurry of investigation into the Strava heatmap when he posted on Twitter about potential US military operations located in Afghanistan and regarding Turkish military in Syria. It wasn't long before other researchers jumped on the bandwagon, identifying European military installations throughout Africa and likely CIA "black" sites. More concerning was the possibility of identifying who was doing the activity.

In the wake of the uproar, the US and other countries revised their regulations about wearable GPS-enabled devices and tracking of activities through websites or apps like Strava or MapMyRun. Pokémon Go had already been banned from use on military phones in 2016 due to similar privacy concerns, although even the Pentagon had a Pokémon "gym" in the building's center courtyard. In the end, both users of these apps and websites and employers need to think about the digital trail people leave behind when using wearable devices and smartphones to track fitness data and the privacy tradeoffs that might be made.

—End Sidebar—

Virtual Reality: Climbing Mount Everest from Your Couch

If you prefer solitary workouts to a group but still want to make sure your yoga poses are correct or that you have the right weightlifting form, virtual reality and smart mirrors might be for you. Smart mirrors offer the personalization of a coach or instructor to correct your form and motivate you to push your workout harder, while giving you instant feedback. Mirror, a New York-based start-up purchased by Lululemon Athletica in June 2020, sells an Internet-connected mirror and offers a variety of workouts, from yoga to high-intensity interval training (HIIT) workouts; Tempo Studio focuses on weight training. When used with a compatible heart rate monitor, some systems can provide real-time feedback for you to pick up your pace or slow it down, and they give you performance metrics at the end of the workout, including estimated calories burned. While they might not quite replace a personal coach, users can feel more confident they are doing an exercise correctly with instant feedback.

Virtual reality (VR) is a relative newcomer to the fitness world. What VR offers to workouts is a truly visually immersive experience. Imagine feeling like you're literally flying over the Alps, diving to the depths of the ocean, or racing against the competition—all the while building your core muscles and balance. You can feel the exhilaration of skiing moguls from the comfort of your climate-controlled living room, or work up a sweat smashing blocks with a light saber to the beat of your favorite tunes, or boxing against Floyd Mayweather.

Early VR platforms required the headset to be tethered to a computer, though that has since been eliminated through the release of all-in-one headsets, like the Oculus Quest in 2019. But VR has been somewhat slow to gain popularity as an exercise platform. After all, the idea of having to wear a somewhat bulky headset while you work up a sweat is less than ideal for most—even if you add in special sweat-catching liners. The number of dedicated workout games is also limited but continues to grow.

What could catapult VR from its techie niche to a more mainstream following? Options include replacing handheld plastic sensors with haptic gloves to provide feedback and resistance, making grasping onto rock ledges or packing a punch more realistic. Another is eliminating the large headset and replacing it with something less obtrusive. Both of these are on the horizon or emerging for a number of manufacturers. And at least one company is betting that you'd be willing to step into a bodysuit to get the most out of your VR workout. The Teslasuit combines haptic feedback (the technology that tricks your brain into thinking you're actually feeling or grabbing something in VR) with biometric monitoring, so you can better track just how many calories that workout actually burned. Finally, most VR games are designed to visually make users feel like they are in the environment, not necessarily make them move around in real life. As demand continues to grow for VR workouts, manufacturers will diversify their offerings. In the next few years, your workout might be a yoga class on the beaches of Bali, where you get instant feedback on your form, or downhill skiing in Switzerland, where Olympic champions like Bode Miller or Lindsey Vonn race you to the finish.

What's for Dinner?

The secret to a healthy lifestyle isn't just exercise— it's also what you're eating. The nearly $14 billion weight-loss market demonstrates just how many of us could use a little help in that area, and where AI can excel.

If you're like most people, the question of what's for dinner is met with dread at the end of a workday. If you're also trying to lose a few pounds or adhere to the keto diet, or you have a houseful of picky eaters, trying to plan healthy meals that meet everyone's requirements can feel like trying to wage peace between warring countries.

Enter Beyoncé. Yes, the Queen Bey herself is using AI to help her fans eat the kinds of vegan meals she eats. With the help of health and wellness guru Marco Borges, Beyoncé and Jay-Z launched a meal-planning app to help users with grocery shopping, recipes, and cooking instructions. It's like a one-stop app for everything food, personalized to the user's preferences. Don't have time to cook large meals during the week but like to experiment on the weekend? Have someone in the household with nut allergies? No problem for this AI-enhanced platform that learns what works for you over time.

While Beyoncé and Jay-Z may be among the most famous to enter the health and wellness arena, they have many competitors, each aiming to help you by making the eating (and shopping and menu planning) part of your weight loss or the healthy eating journey simpler. Heali is a recently launched app that takes AI meal planning one step further. Designed to accommodate thirty different diets, the app also helps users identify possible allergic triggers, or ingredients that can make a condition worse, through natural language processing of nutritional labels and menu items. That's a big help to those of us who have a hard time decoding some of the ingredients on food labels.

Many people use age or event milestones to spur them to eat healthier or get into better shape. In the early 2000s, Mike Lee and his then-fiancée sought the help of a fitness trainer to help them get ready for their upcoming beach wedding. The trainer recommended tracking the number of calories the pair ate daily. At that time, there were no helpful apps to log in meals, so the two had to do it the old-fashioned way—with paper and pencil. Lee decided that there needed to be a better way to track foods and their nutritional content, and in September 2005, the MyFitnessPal website was launched.

Meal tracking is a foundation of many weight loss and health lifestyle plans, including Weight Watchers and Noom. The goal is to have users be more mindful of what they are eating; if you pay more attention to every morsel you put in your mouth, you might make better choices in terms of amounts or kinds of foods you eat. It's a pretty basic concept, but if you've ever tried actually recording literally every piece of food, it can be overwhelming. How can you accurately track your calories or portion size when eating out? And what about recipes you make at home? How do you make sure the nutritional content is right?

This is where apps like MyFitnessPal or FitGenie excel—by making it easier than ever to track your food intake, down to your macros. Many apps now have extensive databases of verified nutritional contents, even for restaurant chains, so you can stay on track even when eating out. What's more, these apps are using AI to make the process even easier, by letting you take a picture of your plate and instantly calculating the calorie and nutrition content.

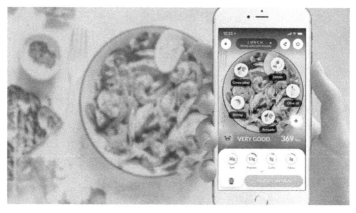

Figure 2.3. AI-enabled meal tracking.
[https://venturebeat.com/2019/11/20/foodvisor-raises-4-5-million-
for-its-ai-driven-app-that-helps-track-what-you-eat/]

Simply point and click and you might find that your dinner plate is a healthy balance of nutrients and clocks in at 725 calories, or maybe that after dinner banana split is a whopping 1,200 calories. By giving users the information without judgment (after all, what if you ran a marathon that day and the banana split fits nicely into your calorie budget?), you can decide if you want to cut your portion size down, add more fruits and vegetables, or indulge in a once-in-a-while treat.

Though you don't need an app to track calories, and meal planning or grocery shopping can be done without the aid of a website, the popularity of these tools shows how useful they are—especially for folks without a lot of time or energy to devote to the tasks in the first place. Like many AI- and machine-learning–based systems, the more data and better training they obtain, the more beneficial people will find them. So in the future, the answer to what's for dinner won't fill you with dread—the answer will be tailored to you, based on the day of the week, the foods you like, and what you already have in the pantry, and it will be at your fingertips.

Too Tired to Sleep

After a long, stressful day, have you ever crawled into bed, certain you'd be asleep before your head hit the pillow, only to lie awake for hours or wake up in the middle of the night and be unable to go back to sleep? Sleep disorders like insomnia are pretty common, affecting about 30 percent of adults, according to the American Academy of Sleep Medicine, and the CDC reports that many of us don't get our recommended hours of sleep regularly. If you fall into these groups, you've got plenty of company and lots of strategies to help. Mindfulness training or meditation is one option that is garnering new interest, due to smartphones and AI.

If you think of meditation, what springs to mind? People sitting cross-legged in the lotus position with their hands resting upturned on their knees while chanting, "Om"? Meditation doesn't require becoming a yogi or seeking a spiritual guru. Research has shown it can reduce feelings of stress, anxiety, and depression, and improve sleep quality. But what if you don't know how to meditate or feel like you can't slow your thoughts down enough to relax? There's an app (and probably dozens!) for that.

Headspace and Calm are two of the oldest and most well-known apps that teach users how to meditate (or practice 'mindfulness') and relax. Soothing voices guide you through meditations to help you get to sleep, fall back asleep, or de-stress you in the middle of a hectic workday. While meditation isn't new, using AI to make it better is.

In 2018, Headspace acquired an AI company to improve the personalization of its meditation app and make it more responsive to users. Instead of generic meditations, the app anticipates users interacting in a more natural way. Stressed out? Simply tell Headspace, and the meditation will help you relax. Can't get to sleep? Tell the app you need to sleep, and it will choose a meditation designed to put you on the road to dreamland. Headspace is far from the only meditation app leveraging the power of AI and machine learning to help people get a better night's sleep or reduce stress and anxiety. Calm, Mindbliss, and Aura are a few more that are taking the ancient practice of meditation and bringing it into the twenty-first century with technology. And while right now you might have to give the app a push in the right direction by telling it how you're feeling, imagine how helpful it would be to have the app automatically sense that you're stressed out, depressed, or angry, and automatically give you the meditation you need.

Ambient music and nature sounds feature prominently in meditation apps, and science is playing a role in determining the most relaxing, sleep-inducing song. British band Marconi Union turned to researchers to help it create a track that could lower blood pressure and heart rate (in turn, lowering stress levels). The result, "Weightless," is a blend of electronica and nature sounds that puts listeners into a zen-like state—ideal for relaxing or falling asleep.

Some people find autonomous sensory meridian response (ASMR) better at reducing stress. Scientists have described ASMR as a tingling sensation across the scalp, neck, or back that occurs after some visual or auditory stimuli. YouTube is full of ASMR videos—with people whispering, passing a soft brush over skin, or popping soap bubbles. The effect is pleasurable, and some believe that it can help induce sleep or deep relaxation. In a recent study, scientists combined ASMR with tones played simultaneously in each ear, producing brain waves that are similar to what happens as you move from being awake to sleep. While the study didn't investigate whether people actually fell asleep, the evidence suggests that if meditation isn't for you, ASMR might help with your insomnia.

Do you toss and turn at night and struggle to get comfortable in bed? Your mattress might be to blame. Once upon a time, beds differed only in the number of coils they had and how fancy their fabric coverings were. Then pillow-top and motorized, adjustable mattresses hit the scene. In recent years, the options grew with the introduction of memory foam mattresses, like Casper and Purple, that come to your home compressed and expand when you take off the cover. The number of mattress options today can make you feel like the princess from the fairy tale *The Princess and the Pea*, trying to find exactly the right one for you.

Wouldn't it be great if your bed could automatically adjust to your sleep needs, from firmness to temperature, based on how frequently you roll over, your heart rate, or how deeply you breathe? Sensors built into some mattresses can do just that. Eight Sleep's beds and companion app provide insight into your sleep patterns and offer suggestions to improve your sleep. If you wake up in the middle of the night, you can turn to the app for a guided meditation designed to put you back to sleep. Sleep Number beds can be paired with some smart devices to identify patterns between quality of sleep and room temperature. ReST beds can adjust automatically, based on feedback from two-thousand pressure points within the mattress. No matter what your mattress preference, companies are integrating advanced technologies to give you a better night's sleep.

Who among us hasn't had to pull up the covers in the middle of the night when we get chilled or have tossed and turned before throwing off the blanket because we get overheated? Many of us, myself included, need our bedrooms and beds to be at the perfect temperature to help us fall asleep and stay asleep. I had the opportunity to chat with Texan Tony Federico about what it's like to actually use a smart bed. Tony calls his smart bed a "game changer."

A self-admitted early adopter of tech, Tony went looking for a solution to bad sleep and found a smart bed. Originally from Michigan, Tony had difficulty falling asleep in the hot, humid Texas summers. Even air conditioning couldn't bring the temperature down low enough for him, and his wife (and his wallet) didn't always appreciate a freezing cold bedroom. A smart mattress seemed like a good compromise.

Tony's mattress looks a lot like any other foam mattress—with a few key differences. In addition to memory foam and sensors built into the mattress, the Eight Sleep mattress adds a thin layer of water contained within a grid on top. Like the waterbeds of yesterday, the water layer conforms to your body, reducing pressure points that cause pain. The similarity stops there, however. The mattress is connected to a device that looks like a large Apple HomePod or Amazon Alexa that houses the "brains" behind the mattress and keeps the water at the right temperature throughout the night. Want to climb into a cozy warm bed in the middle of winter? No problem— the water can heat the bed, making it irresistible to leave. Sleep "hot," like many of us do, tossing the sheets aside in the middle of the night? The Eight Sleep mattress can keep the bed downright chilly. You can set the temperature to the right spot for you (and your partner can do the same for that side of the bed), and the smart mattress will keep you both sleeping happily all night long.

That's what sold Tony on his new bed in the first place—the idea that he (and his wife) could sleep more comfortably without having to keep his air conditioner running on max all summer long. After using the bed for a few months, he said that he started feeling more awake and productive during the day, benefits he credits to sleeping better at night. More than a year later, he's been able to reset his sleep schedule and feel more rested—and he has the data to show for it.

Are You Ready for the Future?

In this chapter, we've seen ways that AI and machine learning are already helping us to be more active and eat healthier. We've seen apps that help us plan meals and share our marathon victories or weight loss with friends, and smart beds and meditation apps that use AI and machine learning to help us get better sleep and reduce our anxiety levels. Where will the future take us?

A few years from now, let's say your annual checkup at the doctor reveals that you've got type 2 diabetes. Your doctor recommends losing about thirty pounds and wants you to exercise more frequently. He or she recommends finding a weight loss app that works for you and walking at least ten thousand steps every day for six months before starting you on medication. This seems pretty consistent with what your doctor might tell you today for the same situation.

But instead of sending you on your way with little follow-up for six months, you download an app that plans all of your meals, from breakfast to dinner and snacks, complete with nutritional information. You won't be stuck eating salad after salad with no end in sight either. By learning the kind of foods you like (and which ones you hate), the app will make sure your menu is filled with a variety of nutritious foods that you'll enjoy and recommend new ones that are sure to please. And when it learns that you prefer to go out to eat or get takeout once or twice a week, it can suggest healthy options to keep you on track while still letting you enjoy the meal. It can also recommend meal delivery options, like HelloFresh or Blue Apron, for nights when you're too busy to cook a meal from scratch. The app will also read data collected from your smartwatch or fitness tracker, so it knows when you've been more active and automatically adjusts the planned meals to accommodate your increased caloric needs—suggesting an extra serving of heart-healthy nuts or fruit, or even a cookie or two.

Your apps will work together too. The meal-planning app might analyze data from your connected scale—adjusting your sodium intake to account for a particularly salty dinner the night before. If you lose the weight too quickly, the app will change your recommendations or weekly meal plan. If you are stuck at the same weight for too long, not only will it shake up your menu, but your fitness tracking app could recommend adding weight training or increasing the number of steps you take each day. After a week of hard workouts that leave you having a difficult time getting comfortable when it's time for bed, your mattress will automatically adjust to cradle you in softness and keep the temperature just perfect for a great night's sleep.

These apps will be able to learn your patterns—so if you're tied to your desk during the week with little time to exercise, they will recommend quick breaks you can do in your office and remind you to stretch during the week periodically to prevent injury on your weekend workouts. And if you're motivated by friendly competition, the app will help you find others of similar ability or health goals. Want to run a marathon? Great—the app will sort you into a group of first-time marathoners, design a practical training plan, and encourage you through both individual and group benchmarks. If a marathon seems impossible, it'll help you go from couch to 5k (a little more than three miles) or even just around the block. When you're done working out and ready for bed, your mattress with help ease the aches and pains from training, and your meditation app will have you asleep in no time. And to make it all even easier, the most you'll have to do is download the apps, link them to the other accounts/apps/wearables, and go.

Taking Control of the Future—Now

As this chapter has shown you, we are almost at the scenario I just described. Some of the technology to turn this into reality already exists or is close to production. The Apple Watch (see Chapter Three) is a case in point for wearables and fitness training, while apps like MyFitnessPal are edging closer to making nutrition as seamless and convenient for users as possible. Even when we can't get to the gym, working out can mirror the competition through apps and virtual reality—complete with real-time feedback from virtual coaches. What can you do now?

1. Try downloading an app, like Strava or Garmin (if you use a Garmin fitness tracker) and join a virtual challenge or two. Compete against your friends or other users around the world as you get into shape or train for your next race.

2. Need to lose weight? There are subscription-based programs (like Weight Watchers or Noom) as well as free apps to help you track your calories and suggest healthy meals. If you tried counting calories or macros before and were frustrated by the clunky user interface, you may be pleasantly surprised by new AI-enhanced technology that lets you simply take a picture of your food.

3. Feel stressed all the time or plagued by insomnia? If working out doesn't always fit your schedule, try meditation as a way to clear your mind and install some calm into your busy day or before bed. With meditation apps embracing AI to be more responsive to your needs and adding features like ASMR, you're sure to find an app that meets your needs. And if you want a more comfortable, data-driven night's sleep, a smart mattress might change your life.

4. If you don't get motion sickness, VR workouts may be the next best thing to get you sweaty in no time. VR platforms like Oculus Go that don't require you to be tethered to a computer and gorgeous visualizations are second only to being there in person. VR could be for you if the idea of yoga on a beach in Bali or mastering the sword in a gladiator arena sounds like fun.

CHAPTER THREE:

THE DOCTOR IS IN YOUR DEVICE

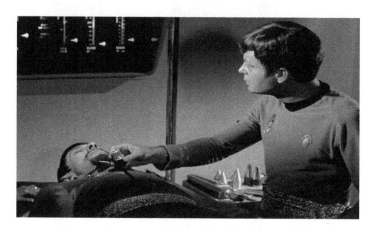

Star Trek was ahead of its time in many ways, and not just because the sci-fi franchise portrayed a future several centuries after the series first aired in the 1960s. The cult classic TV show/films foresaw what life might be like in the twenty-third century, when humankind would be hurtling on spaceships through unknown universes. Much of the show was fantasy, of course, but the series has been heralded for foreshadowing the future with uncanny accuracy. Dozens of articles have appeared on the topic, even one in the venerable *Scientific American*. Many tech writers have credited the show with anticipating and even inspiring the advent of myriad of modern technologies, including iPads, flat-screen TVs, Bluetooth headsets, Google Glass, sliding doors, and chatbots like Siri that can answer our questions and complete tasks.

But perhaps no technology imagined by *Star Trek* has enticed more international interest than the medical tricorder. The device, which resembled a clunky transistor radio on the original show, included a small, detachable scanner that Dr. McCoy, Spock, or other *Enterprise* crew member could use to instantly diagnose the health of a human or Vulcan alike. The magical medical tricorder then pushed the patient's clinical information to a master databank, allowing intergalactic doctors to learn more about all life to help further hone the technology. As I'm about to explain, we aren't as far off from this scenario as you might think!

Since the tricorder's first appearance, the device has inspired endless intrigue, spurring both techies and Trekkies to try to recreate the tool for real-life use. The technology needed to devise a modern-day tricorder, however, has long lagged behind the enthusiasm to do so. In 2014, telecom giant Qualcomm hoped to speed the science along, launching a global competition called the Qualcomm Tricorder XPRIZE and offering $10 million to anyone who could create a tricorder that diagnosed thirteen different medical conditions and monitored five vital signs, all independent of a physician. Qualcomm's intent was to give people control over their own healthcare—a theme of patient empowerment that you'll see associated with many AI-enabled medical machines.

Eight international teams were selected to show off their prototype tricorders and compete for the $7 million grand prize. Although none were completely successful in meeting the competition's demands, several came close, and the XPRIZE Foundation awarded more than $3 million to the top-scoring two teams and an additional $100,000 "Bold Epic Innovator" award to a third, donating more than $5 million of the remaining original purse to ongoing efforts in consumer testing and adaption of tricorders for hospital use in developing nations. In the four years since the conclusion of the Tricorder XPRIZE competition, the teams have met with varied success in moving their technologies from prototype to consumer-ready.

The "Bold Epic Innovator" team from Canada is arguably one of the most successful. Cloud DX had its beginnings in the aftermath of a devasting 2010 earthquake in Haiti. Physician Sonny Kohli was volunteering and realized quickly the need for a small, portable device that could help doctors diagnose patients. Just a few years later, back in Ontario, Kohli joined forces with others who would later become the Cloud DX team. Cloud DX's tricorder, named Vitaliti, continuously monitored multiple vital signs, including blood pressure, heart rate, blood oxygen saturation, and temperature.

Cloud DX today has made significant strides in tackling the problem of monitoring and diagnosing patients, inside and outside of the hospital. Its Connected Health Kit can do a lot of what its tricorder could do: monitor blood pressure, temperature, weight, glucose, and blood oxygen levels. For doctors looking to keep an eye on patients who are discharged from the hospital, or in settings where hospital care is difficult to come by, the Connected Health Kit addresses many concerns. In the next chapter, you'll see how devices like this one are an integral part of the future of healthcare. Tools like tricorders may seem like science fiction, and it's true that we're not (yet) able to wave a tiny device over the length of someone's body and one second later know absolutely everything about their health condition. But Cloud DX and companies like it are showing us that science fiction is well on its way to becoming reality.

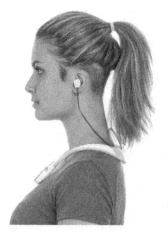

Figure 3.1. CloudDx Vitaliti XPrize Tricorder Device.
[https://www.clouddx.com/#/vitality]

Empowering the Patient: How the Smartphone Is Transforming Medicine

Mobile health isn't new. The practice of using personal mobile devices like smartphones with wearable sensors like watches to track and even diagnose medical conditions has been around for more than a decade. The Withings company launched its connected body scale in June 2009 and its blood pressure monitor (connected to the iPhone) in 2011, for example. And Apple made its foray into tracking personal fitness and health when it teamed up with Nike in 2006 with the Nike+iPod Sports Kit.

What is new, however, is the breadth of today's technology. In the past several years, AI has advanced so rapidly that smartphone apps and their connected sensors can now accomplish feats previously inconceivable just several years ago. Using only a smartphone, you can now prevent health emergencies, diagnose clinical disorders, and even treat conditions without prescription drugs.

AI isn't the only technology driving the breakneck explosion of mobile medicine either. AI-enabled software is only as good as the data it relies on to make medical predictions. Today, software companies have more data than they've ever had before, thanks to millions of users worldwide who've been tracking their heart rate, steps, sleep, and other biometrics, knowingly or not, for years. This ever-expanding databank allows software manufacturers to hone the accuracy of their existing apps while creating new software and sensors that can monitor, diagnose, and treat people in other amazing, new ways.

Another factor fueling the transformation of smartphone medicine is hardware, which has become more sophisticated in recent years. This hardware upgrade has given our phones the ability to process and store more data in a smaller space, making it as powerful as some supercomputers. Today's smartphone even outshines the supercomputer found on the spaceship Orion, launched by

NASA in 2014 to prepare for man's first crewed mission to Mars.

As our smartphones get smarter—and our out-of-pocket healthcare costs continue to rise—the world of medical apps has exploded. Today, there are more than three hundred fifty thousand different healthcare apps, and the mobile-health market is expected to approach $290 billion in revenue by 2025. It's a fascinating contradiction: while the costs of technology continue to drop (does anyone remember how expensive the first personal computers were?), healthcare costs keep rising. It's not really surprising that there's a lot of interest, especially from big tech and the business world, in using the power of technology to tackle one of healthcare's biggest challenges—cost. I believe that's one of the reasons we've seen so many tech companies enter the healthcare and life sciences industries; their outsider point of view is not unlike the one I had looking in at the telecom industry and imagining how GPS could be used in a whole new way. The industry is revolutionizing not only how we look at medicine, but also the power we hold in our hands to take care of our own health.

Think about it for a moment. If you could own an app that could diagnose you with the same accuracy as your primary care provider, you'd have the virtual equivalent of an on-call physician with you at all times who could help streamline your care in real life. Earache? Let the AI-enabled app, maybe combined with access to a telehealth provider, distinguish between something that needs an office visit in the next day or two, a simple prescription with advice to follow up in a week, or a recommendation to head to the emergency room or urgent care right away. Without the cost or chaos of an unnecessary office or urgent visit, you'd be able to consult this virtual physician regularly without waiting to get seriously sick to realize something was wrong with you—or if you should just take an over-the-counter pain reliever and rest for the day.

Similarly, if your phone and a few connected sensors could monitor your blood pressure, cholesterol, and other basic biomarkers around the clock, you'd know within seconds if something was irregular rather than waiting to reach the same conclusion after developing symptoms.

How many of us head to the dermatologist every year for a head-to-toe exam to look for signs of skin cancer? What if your phone could also scan your skin for signs of cancer or other ailments without the yearly trip, and in the comfort of your own home? And then transmit the scan to the dermatologist's office, where it could be looked over? If things look good, you might get a letter in your electronic health record saying you're good for another six months or a year. If the dermatologist sees something concerning, you might get a phone call instead, asking you to schedule an appointment for a follow-up in office. The setup could also be ideal for parents who are worried about a rash on their child. You'd have the ability to know what was wrong, probably in less time and at a lower cost than it takes to get an accurate diagnosis today. In short, smartphones are democratizing medicine in ways we've never seen before—an idea first touted by the eminent cardiologist Dr. Eric Topol in his 2014 book *The Patient Will See You Now*. Since then, more of us own smartphones. Nearly four billion worldwide, including 81 percent of US adults, possess this portable supercomputer. Now, anyone who has a smartphone or smartwatch can potentially access quality healthcare, no matter how old they are or where they live, whether in a big city with access to excellent hospitals and specialists or in a rural area without many medical facilities or qualified physicians. We'll still need trained doctors, of course, and there's some level of infrastructure needed to get healthcare systems ready to receive data from our phones and digital devices, but the smartphone has become medicine's great equalizer, making it easier for everyone to obtain top medical attention, regardless of their nationality, ethnicity, age, income level, insurance coverage, or other factors that have traditionally limited quality healthcare.

Sidebar:
The New Power Struggle: How Smartphone Medicine Is Making Tech Companies the New Kings of Healthcare

Empowering patients to take care of their health by using their smartphones is upending the medical industry too. While hospitals, doctors' offices, and other healthcare facilities have traditionally hoarded patient data, software companies are now collecting that information—and, depending on the popularity of their apps, amassing much more of it.

The data owned by software companies can also be more comprehensive than what many doctors and hospitals have. While physicians and clinics collect data on you whenever you go in for a checkup or have a health emergency, apps can track your biometrics around the clock, or as long as you leave your device powered on.

In the new age of AI, where data is more precious than oil, the more information you have, the more powerful you become. Companies like Apple and Google are using their massive databanks to expand into healthcare with innovative products like watches that administer electrocardiograms, but they are also sharing the information with medical institutions and scientists, helping to influence and contribute to the conversation on medical research. You can even carry around your medical records (or at least some part of them) on your phone.

For example, Apple enrolls thousands of users in clinical studies via its apps, Apple Watch, and a software platform called ResearchKit. Perhaps the best-known example of Apple's foray into research is the Apple Heart Study, a virtual trial that included more than four hundred thousand participants recruited through the Apple Watch's heart rate app. In 2019, in an article published in the prestigious *New England Journal of Medicine*, the study concluded that 84 percent of people who received irregular pulse notifications were, in fact, experiencing atrial fibrillation, and that the notification prompted more than half to seek medical attention.

Similarly, Alphabet, the parent company of Google, collects data for scientific research with Verily Study Watch through its life sciences company Verily, and studies human longevity and anti-aging in Calico Labs. Microsoft, IBM, and Intel all partner with universities and other research outlets to leverage their technology, databanks, and brands into medical science.

You might wonder why these tech companies are working with universities or others doing research. After all, the data is the data, right? Not so fast. Remember my GPS idea that went nowhere because I was a life sciences guy and that was a tech problem (at the time)? In some ways, healthcare is still pretty siloed. With the stakes so high, we are talking about human lives, after all—doctors and researchers want to make sure the information is accurate.

Healthcare providers and regulating bodies want to see data showing that something works—ideally in the context of a clinical trial. For example, if a patient were to come to his or her doctor with a spreadsheet export of heart rate data, the doctor probably wouldn't know what to do with it. The doctor would want to know where it came from, how accurate the reading was, and how it correlated with the activity the patient was doing at the time. Getting all of that might mean downloading data from several different apps on the patient's phone and wearables. It would be a challenge for the doctor to make sense of all of that data, and in the end, the doctor would probably still want to see the results of a clinical trial before making new treatment decisions.

Companies like Evidation Health are one answer to that. Evidation, a company I was involved with at its inception, works with pharmaceutical and technology companies to collect that information from millions of people—real-world evidence—and make sense of the data. Using "digital" trials, the company has published scientific papers on the effectiveness of app-driven education and management of glucose levels in people with type 2 diabetes and constipation, and the differences in patient-reported symptoms and biomarkers, like heart rate in patients with flu and COVID-19.

For megatech companies like Apple and Google, healthcare isn't the primary revenue stream; it's just gravy on the metaphorical bird of their business model. This gives tech titans leeway to create inroads into healthcare without having to answer to investors or make ends meet in order to pay their employees. On the consumer side of the equation, it can mean that the devices, software, or other products they create might be less expensive, without a huge markup for profit. For smaller software companies, big tech giants like Apple have created a safe space for start-ups to develop apps and for entrepreneurs to manufacture connected devices. Whether empowering tech to control the future of our health is a good thing or not, only time will tell.

The Details Before the Download

Your smartphone can be a powerful medical device if you want it to be. But like any medical tool or treatment, there are caveats and concerns that come with it.

If you believe you're suffering from a medical condition, whether your phone confirms it or not, see a doctor or other medical specialist. Not all apps are designed to diagnose—some are simply intended to guide or alert you when you might need medical attention.

What's more, not all apps are approved by the FDA, either because the government doesn't consider it a medical device, or the app hasn't completed enough clinical testing to meet FDA guidelines. However, many apps that haven't been approved by the FDA might still help improve your health; it's best to approach them with a modicum of caution. As you might imagine, with dozens of new apps hitting the various app stores every week, this is a rapidly evolving space.

Finally, before using any app as a diagnostic device, check with your doctor or other healthcare provider. I'm not a healthcare provider, and the information in this book is designed to inform you about the possibilities—not direct you on how to manage your specific health conditions.

—End Sidebar—

A Dozen (or So) Ways to Improve Your Health Using Your Smartphone

Today, you can find a smartphone app for nearly every medical condition or outcome. Apps abound to monitor heart rate, blood pressure, blood sugar, cholesterol, fertility, sleep, and even brain-wave activity. Some apps can diagnose or offer medical guidance; others share your information with a physician or other healthcare provider. There are apps that mimic medical equipment, turning your smartphone into a digital stethoscope, blood-pressure cuff, thermometer, spirometer, and even ultrasound. You can use your phone to access your electronic health records or connect instantly with a physician via video or text. Your phone can help you find and enroll in a clinical trial or help you shop around for the best price on prescription drugs. With the help of a smartphone and some sensors, you can find out if your child has an ear infection or learn how to walk again after a devastating spinal-cord injury.

In addition to offering innovative ways to let you take control your health, what these apps all have in common is that they're powered by AI and big data.

Simply put, AI comes into the picture in two ways. First, your health data is detected and compiled through the intelligent features of your devices in ways previously not possible, such as heart rate, blood pressure, sleep restlessness, temperature, etc. Second, these smartphone apps can build extremely large data sets across the entire population that uses that app (big data) as well as pulling in outside data from other studies or research related to the same health metrics. This is where AI comes in. When you put these two types of information together and use sophisticated algorithms to identify patterns and see correlations, you can make sense of what's going on with large groups of people, and how health or metrics among populations are changing. You can also tell individual users how their patterns compare to those of others, how their own pattern might change day to day—or in the case of a crisis, diagnose an emergency. But making those connections between individuals and populations only becomes possible with advanced AI tools and software trained to "learn" about patterns and compare them to known healthcare standards.

Data, on the other hand, is the information that these algorithms run on, allowing the apps to learn what's right or wrong with you, based on large data sets created from everyone using these apps.

To apply a very apt analogy, think of AI as the physician—the one who takes your vitals, conducts an exam, and makes a diagnosis. A doctor couldn't do any of this without data, which, in this analogy, is equivalent to years in medical school and real-life experience seeing and treating patients.

All this leads us to the same conclusion: The smartphone undoubtedly sitting within arm's reach of you right now is a tool you can use, if you choose, to improve your health with just a few clicks.

What exactly can your phone do for your health? Here are several ways your phone can improve your health for some common conditions. All the apps mentioned in this section are available for download today and are medical apps. (For smart software that optimizes nutrition, exercise, weight-loss goals, mood, and other wellness aspects, see Chapter Two):

Prevent a heart attack with your watch: The Apple Watch wasn't intended to save lives, but that's exactly what it's doing, thanks to an AI-enabled feature that provides users with an electrocardiogram (ECG) and continuous heartbeat measurement. There are now dozens of stories of how this Apple Watch feature has prevented an untimely death. A woman in Alabama, for example, credits her watch with alerting her that her heart wasn't beating properly—even though she felt fine. Days later, she underwent open-heart surgery. There's also the Seattle man whose watch told him his heart rhythm was irregular, despite normal ECGs whenever he visited the doctor. His physician corroborated the report and prescribed the man blood thinners, preventing stroke. Outside of Apple Watch, apps like KardiaMobile offer accurate ECG readings by using a connected fingertip pad. There are also standalone apps like Cardiio, developed by scientists at MIT, which interpret your heart's electrical activity by analyzing facial-light reflection from a selfie snapped by your phone. By capturing all of the heart rate data from an individual and then comparing it to what is considered "normal," or "abnormal," these AI systems can learn to identify patterns of atrial fibrillation, dropped heartbeats, or other heart rhythm problems, and then alert the patient to see a doctor.

Find out if you're depressed with the app that screens your calls: While it may sound like something only anxious parents do, CompanionMX screens your calls and texts to determine whether you're suffering from depression. The app uses voice recognition to determine whether you have low energy or other signs of depression. Since emotions vary from person to person, CompanionMX relies only on clinical symptoms. Other mental-health apps like Mindstrong work similarly, analyzing how you tap, type, and scroll on your phone to ascertain whether you might be battling depression or a similar mood disorder.

Learn in less than a minute if a mole is melanoma: The app SkinVision may be better at diagnosing skin cancer than dermatologists, according to research. The AI-enabled app, which analyzes a selfie of the suspicious spot in thirty seconds to tell you whether you're low or high risk for developing melanoma, has a 95 percent accuracy rate, beating the 61–66 percent sensitivity of general practitioners and 75–92 percent sensitivity of dermatologists. Still, some health organizations question whether SkinVision can really provide accurate diagnoses or will miss cases of cancer. While the company looks to hone its software and win FDA approval, other outlets are building apps that would allow a telehealth doctor to diagnose a selfie of your mole sent virtually.

Sidebar:
AI Saved My Life: The Watch That Called 911 for a Fallen Cyclist

Doomsday Hill is one of the steepest streets in all of Spokane, Washington, a site of reckoning for thousands of cyclists and runners who negotiate the storied slope every year. For Bob Burdett, Doomsday wasn't his comeuppance, but his kismet.

On a dry day in September, Burdett was riding his bike down Doomsday to Riverside State Park, where he planned to meet his son, Gabe, for a father-son cycling foray. The sixty-three-year-old had already attacked the hill from the other side, crested it, and was zooming back down the backside of the beast. That's the last thing he remembers. "Everything was black and white coming down the hill," Burdett says. "I only knew I took a turn at twenty miles per hour because my Apple Watch was tracking my ride."

Twenty minutes later, Burdett woke up in the back of an ambulance, as paramedics rushed him to a hospital. He was bleeding profusely and had lost consciousness. At the hospital, the doctors told him what had happened: He'd fallen off his bike, was knocked cold, and it was his Apple Watch that dialed 911, not a passerby, after it detected Burdett hadn't moved for more than a minute.

The feature, available on Apple Watch Series 4 and later models, uses AI algorithms to sense when someone has taken a hard fall. When a fall occurs, the watch starts sending you alerts and sounding an audible alarm, which you can cancel if all is OK. But if all's not OK, the alarm grows louder, alerting others in the area. If nothing occurs within a minute, the watch calls 911, sharing your location with emergency services as longitude and latitude coordinates. The watch also notifies a family member or friend.

"I never knew whether the detection app worked, but I do a lot of riding on my own, and I figured it was a way to be responsible for myself," says Burdett, an experienced cyclist. "I was utterly stunned when it worked."

Riding alone at a time when Doomsday had little pedestrian or vehicular traffic, Burdett might have remained on the side of the road for however long, unconscious, bleeding, and quickly fading, Instead, his watch dialed 911 at a time when every minute mattered—and it also notified Gabe, who immediately started searching for his father, only to discover he was already being treated at the hospital.

Later that evening, Burdett was released from the hospital with a concussion and a few stiches over his eye. Within weeks, his story was picked up by Seattle media and went viral.

"I've been emailed and notified by people all over the world—tons of people have requested my friendship on Facebook," he says. "They tell me that they wanted to get their parents an Apple Watch to make sure they don't fall, and this finally inspired them to do it. I highly recommend it."

Only one week after his accident, Burdett was back on his bike—with his Apple Watch.

"I was sold on the Apple Watch before it proved itself," Burdett says. "But now, I won't leave home without it. Honestly, I wear it every day."

Conduct a urinalysis in your bathroom: The dreaded doctor's office pee test: you never have to go at the right time and it's always … awkward. Apps like Dip.io are obviating the inconvenience by allowing your phone to perform urinalyses in the privacy of your own home. The analytic app provides a urine cup for you to pee in, and with the help of a disposable dipstick and courtesy a smartphone photo, Dip.io matches the color of your urine to its databank of dipsticks to determine whether your kidneys are functioning normally, or if you have a urinary-tract infection.

Take away chronic pain without surgery or prescription drugs: The quest to solve chronic pain in America has traditionally revolved around two options—prescription drugs and surgery, which don't always improve patient outcomes. Today, AI is offering an effective alternative that's less invasive and doesn't carry the complications or risks that prescription painkillers do. AppliedVR eases chronic pain from conditions like treatment-resistant fibromyalgia and intractable lower back pain. These are conditions that don't respond to conventional treatment, leaving those patients to suffer. AppliedVR's EaseVRx uses virtual reality (VR) to guide patients with chronic pain through its cognitive behavioral therapy (CBT) immersive program. In a clinical trial comparing the EaseVRx to nature content delivered through the VR headset, EaseVRx was shown to reduce pain intensity and improve activity, mood, and stress in users.

Get a medical exam from the comfort of your couch: It's a common occurrence: Your child wakes up with a fever and sore throat, and you have no clue whether it's strep, tonsillitis, or the flu. But instead of rushing him or her to the pediatrician, you use TytoCare, which connects you via video with a doctor who can diagnose and prescribe a treatment plan for your child on the spot. The doctor performs a virtual medical exam using TytoCare's connected sensors, which can take temperature and heart rate, provide digital sounds of the heart and lungs, and snap high-quality images and videos of the ears, throat, and skin. Not just for upper respiratory issues, the app can also diagnose bites, rashes, stomach pain, and ear infections.

Prevent asthma attacks before they occur: Most people with asthma don't use their inhalers properly, either missing doses or not taking the medication correctly, increasing the risk of attacks and hospitalizations. Propeller Health eradicates these issues by using a sensor that attaches to an inhaler, letting you and your doctor know exactly when and how well you use the device. The app also monitors weather, pollution, and allergens in your area to alert you to know when you're at greater risk for breathing difficulties.

Stop migraine pain with a wearable sensor: Next time you get a migraine, you may want to try Nerivio Migra, an app that connects with an armband to send electrical pulses that can stop your pounding pain. The app, named one of Time magazine's Top 100 Inventions of 2019, relieves two-thirds of all users' pain in two hours or less, according to studies. The distinction of the most popular headache app goes to Migraine Buddy, which claims to have more digital downloads than any other migraine app worldwide. Migraine Buddy tracks potential triggers like weather patterns and what you eat to help you or your physician identify what's causing your migraine pain and how to stop it. The app also includes a virtual support group where users can share stories and tips.

Prevent a fatal drug overdose: Every day, one hundred and thirty Americans die from what may be the US's most preventable problem: drug overdose. But getting help for an overdose doesn't happen easily, as friends or family members usually only discover loved one hours or even days after any hope of resuscitation has passed. That's why researchers at the University of Washington have developed Second Chance, a smartphone app that can detect when someone has overdosed by monitoring his or her breathing. Users anonymously turn on the app whenever they want, prompting the AI-enabled platform to start transmitting sonar waves. The app then interprets how these sound waves bounce off a person's chest to ascertain whether he or she is breathing. If the app doesn't discover a respiratory response, it will automatically dial a friend, physician, or 911.

Monitor your blood sugar 24/7: If you're the one of every ten Americans who suffers from diabetes, you already know the inconvenience that comes with sticking yourself with needles multiple times per day to measure your blood glucose levels. The drill isn't just laborious, but also inconclusive, providing patients with only a snapshot of their blood sugar at any particular time, even though glucose levels can fluctuate quickly. Smartphone apps like Dexcom help diabetics stay safe while eradicating the trouble of traditional blood glucose meters. Instead of using needles, Dexcom relies on a small sensor placed just under the skin that monitors blood glucose continuously, providing up to 288 readings in twenty-four hours. Not just for diabetics, the app is also popular with low-carb dieters, who use it to assess how certain foods affect their individual blood sugar, helping them better control this risk factor for weight gain. And it's been rumored that a new version of the Apple Watch will have the ability to track blood sugar noninvasively.

Assess how healthy you are whenever, wherever you want: Apple's Health app, which now comes preinstalled on every iPhone, has come a long way since it first launched in 2014. Today, the app can track many of the same biometrics your doctor checks during an annual physical, including heart rate, blood pressure, body weight, cholesterol, hydration, menstruation, sleep patterns, and blood glucose. The platform also encourages users to set up a medical ID, which allows first responders to assess personal medical information like blood type, allergies, and preexisting health conditions that can be critical to survival in the event of a medical emergency.

Find out how much oxygen is in your blood: Before the coronavirus outbreak, at-home pulse oximeters were primarily used by pulmonary patients, pilots, and elite athletes in order to get an idea of how much oxygen was in their blood. Blood oxygen levels can indicate how well you're recovering from a respiratory illness, whether you're able to withstand the low-oxygen conditions of high-altitude flights, or how conditioned you are for athletic competition. During the coronavirus pandemic, however, sales of pulse oximeter apps skyrocketed, as Americans looked for ways to monitor COVID-19's respiratory symptoms at home. Apple integrated oxygen saturation reading into its Apple Watch. Digital device manufacturer Masimo, for example, was consistently sold out of its MightySat app after media stars like CNN's Chris Cuomo and SiriusXM host Andy Cohen credited oximeters with helping them track their respiratory health while sick with the virus. Masimo, which also makes FDA-approved pulse oximeter apps for hospital use, pairs MightySat with a fingertip sensor to provide a more accurate blood-oxygen reading than standalone apps deliver.

—End Sidebar—

Cured by Clicking: How Your Smartphone Can Treat You Too

Smartphone apps don't just monitor and diagnose—they can treat conditions too. Digital therapeutics are AI-enabled apps that act like prescription drugs to help treat disease. The apps, which require FDA approval, are backed by reams of research and clinical testing, and are usually available only by prescription. Digital therapeutics are noninvasive, don't carry the side effects many pharmaceuticals do, and have become popular for treating conditions often poorly addressed by traditional medicine, including mental health disorders and neurodegenerative diseases.

Pear Therapeutics, for example, makes several different prescription products available for the smartphone. Its Somryst app helps patients with chronic insomnia overcome the condition by undergoing CBT, a treatment that can be difficult to find in some areas across the country. Those who receive the digital treatment, which is based on AI-driven algorithms, are able to fall asleep faster and stay there without relying on prescription hypnotics like Ambien, which can cause dependency and serious side effects. Similarly, Pear Therapeutics' reSET app provides CBT to those struggling with substance abuse issues. The company is also partnering with drug manufacturer Novartis to develop apps that can treat schizophrenia and multiple sclerosis.

BlueStar, the first-ever FDA-approved digital therapeutic, is a prescription-only app designed to help diabetics manage the disease. The app provides an all-in-one digital diary, tracking daily diet, blood glucose levels, physical activity, and medication intake, which it can also share with a user's healthcare team.

One of the most interesting digital therapeutics to hit the market is an app called LookBack, which uses a virtual-reality headset to let patients with dementia "revisit" any location in the world in the hope of triggering memories. Another therapeutic in the cognitive space is MedRhythms, which pairs with shoe sensors and headphones to help people with Parkinson's disease, multiple sclerosis, brain injuries, and other neurodegenerative conditions improve their gait and balance. The app does this by analyzing information from shoe sensors, then cuing music shown to stimulate areas of the brain that can improve motor coordination.

The Future of Smartphone Medicine: Swiping Up on Tomorrow's Technology

Picture the year 2030. Where are you? What do you look like? And what does your smartphone look like? If the futurists are right, your smartphone may be a hologram projected onto your hand or in front of your face, emitted from a small ring or bracelet that contains only nanoscopic hardware. There will be no ports or wires, and your phone's camera technology will be absolutely breathtaking. In fact, what we think of as a smartphone today might really just be a smart device—able to do everything our phones can do and more.

Wearables and other sensors that connect with our phones will also look and function differently. For starters, sensors will be smarter, as AI technology continues to improve and companies amass more data, increasing the accuracy and diagnostic capabilities of their analytic software. Glasses and contact lenses will not only fix your eyesight but also let you know when you need to drink more water, or encourage you to take a stretching break at work, help you read email when you're away from your desk, give you step-by-step directions to a restaurant, or even translate street signs and menus when you're in a foreign country.

Connected sensors will be smaller and nimbler, and the software running them faster than we can imagine right now, so much so that they will be part of us, inside our clothing and contact lenses, as well as inside of us, as tiny implantable or ingestible microchips. In short, the future of smartphone medicine may just blur the boundary between man and machines.

Here's a look at what smartphone medicine might look like tomorrow, as it continues to empower you to take control of your own health:

Electronic tattoos: Your ink options tomorrow are going to look a lot different from today's tattooed names, geometric designs, and dark-blue dedications to loved ones. Electronic tattoos adhere to skin like temporary tattoos, but are much more sophisticated, with the ability to provide continuous information to your phone about your respiratory rate, hydration levels, blood sugar, your heart's electrical activity, and other biometrics. Made from smart fabrics or hydrogels and tiny electrodes that attach directly to skin, e-tattoos promise to deliver more accurate data than whatever can be collected using a wearable sensor on your wrist, including the ability to wear multiple sensors at the same time. Some companies are also trying to develop digital tattoos that would deliver medication via your smartphone, which would control the dosage amount and time.

Implantables: Why wear a sensor when you can have one implanted, capable of continuously communicating what's going on inside you with incredible accuracy? While implantables already exist—Eversense, for example, makes an implant that sits just under your skin to monitor blood sugar—the technology is expanding in incredible ways. Perhaps one of the most outrageous new concepts comes from supermind Elon Musk, who is working on a set of implants called Neuralink that would allow paralyzed patients to control their phones or computers with their thoughts. In the more realistic future, implantables may let you track via your phone your heart activity, cholesterol, temperature, internal pH, and even the medicines you take.

Similar to digital tattoos, implantables could also deliver drugs through an app. A company backed by the Bill and Melinda Gates Foundation, for example, is developing an implantable chip that would dispense birth control whenever you want it. And while it's been in the works for some time, tech companies hope to debut implantable sensors that would allow you or your doctor to obtain your medical records by simply scanning your implant with a smartphone app.

Ingestibles: Companies like Medtronic are already making swallowable pills with cameras that help doctors monitor conditions like gastrointestinal cancers or stomach ulcers. But the wide world of biosensors is growing beyond surveillance, as scientists develop ways ingestible devices can monitor medication adherence, diagnose, and even treat medical conditions. For example, researchers are working on ingestible sensors that assess the health of the body's microbiome, a community of trillions of bacteria and other organisms in our gut that influences nearly every aspect of our physical and mental health. Other ingestible sensor ideas include smart pills that can sense conditions inside the body for up to a month and deliver drugs via a smartphone app in the right dose at the right time.

Smart clothing: Smart fabrics already exist. The company Nanowear, for example, manufactures base layers with miniscule sensors stitched in to allow doctors to monitor patients' heart function through a smartphone app. Now the company wants to empower patients at home by developing sleep shirts that would predict if and when they might experience a traumatic heart event. Other smart fabrics are in the works, including bras that monitor heart rate or can identify potential cancers, stockings that track leg swelling, clothing that raises or lowers body temperature, and pants that can help older people walk with better balance. More e-textile projects include T-shirts that alleviate back pain, belly bands that monitor a developing fetus, and shirts that shock you if you start to have a serious heart problem.

Smart contact lenses: Today, forty-five million Americans wear contact lenses. But many more of us might wear an unperceivable slice of plastic if it helped prevent, diagnose, and treat disease. Smart contact lenses are already used by some ophthalmologists. The company Sensimed, for example, makes a lens that allows eye doctors to monitor patients continuously for signs of glaucoma. But the smart lenses of tomorrow will include more functions, as companies devise ways to pack thousands of biosensors into individual lenses engineered to pick up early indicators of disease. A company in South Korea, for example, already has a blueprint for a lens that can continuously monitor blood glucose, letting diabetics manage their medication through a connected smartphone app.

Hearables: Forget about wearables and say hello to their sexier sister. The field of hearables, which includes AI-enabled headphones, earbuds, and hearing aids, is evolving quickly, as researchers look for more accurate ways to track heart rate, blood pressure, temperature, and even brain-wave activity through ear devices that come connected to smartphone apps. Soon, our AirPods may be able to not only make calls from our phones if we fall but take the place of our hearing aids entirely. Our hearing aids may act like virtual assistants, warning us when our hearts aren't functioning well and reminding us to take our medication. In the near future, hearables may also be able to monitor our stress levels, cuing up calming music when we need it or connecting with nearby thermostats and lighting controls to change our surroundings to a more relaxing setting.

Camera diagnosis: Smartphone apps with sensory devices will continue to proliferate in the future, becoming more adept at alerting us to potential illness and diagnosing medical conditions days, weeks, and even months before we get sick. Part of this improving diagnostic power will come from machine vision, which uses AI to enable computers to see as well as we do. Cameras in our smartphones will also have sharper resolution and more megapixels, allowing a simple selfie to detect everything from anemia to pancreatic cancer. New camera technology may also turn the simple smartphone into a powerful, lab-quality microscope, capable of examining blood cells and identifying potentially harmful pathogens wherever we go.

Chatbots: Whether you know it or not, you've likely been using chatbots for several years. Chatbots are simply software programs that allow you to have a conversation with a computer. Examples include pop-up boxes for virtual assistants online and platforms like Siri, Alexa, and Echo that emulate audible conversation. In healthcare, chatbots will ascertain what's wrong with you by asking about your symptoms and collating data from wearable, implantable, or ingestible sensors. After the chatbot narrows down a possible diagnosis, it can route you to the right doctor, who may see you virtually via video or by text. If your problem is psychological, the chatbot might suggest therapy with another virtual assistant. While some may bemoan the absence of human interaction in these scenarios, the idea of chatbots is gaining more ground, especially in psychological settings, where patients may be too embarrassed to discuss mental or emotional health issues with a real-life therapist or need more daily guidance than one person can provide.

The Future You

Are you seeing your smartphone in a new light? Thinking about downloading a few new apps? It's not difficult to imagine a future, even one just a few years from now, where our phones do the heavy lifting on nearly all of our health and wellness needs combined with a few smart devices or clothes. A time when we could monitor most common biocharacteristics, from weight and height to whether we're getting enough oxygen or if we have a kidney infection. A time when our doctors can get this information securely sent to them through our medical records (which will interface with the data from our apps) and reach out to us when they see concerning trends or will be able to diagnose us faster because we already have some of the basic data they need.

I think we're about halfway to that future time. What isn't clear is just how long it will take us to move from this point of collecting and finding patterns in the data, to one where we (and our healthcare providers) are actively using those patterns to make accurate predictions about our health. For example, it's one thing to use an app to track your migraine headaches. Still another to have the app use analytics to find patterns in the data (does it correspond to nights when you've traveled on a plane or eaten a specific kind of food?). And yet another layer of complexity of AI is to get a notification from the app that suggests you take an earlier flight if possible or pick a restaurant that doesn't use MSG in its food prep (if that's one of your migraine triggers).

So what does this mean for you, today? That answer lies in how much control you want to take, a little bit about how tech-savvy you are, and how comfortable you are with sharing your data. The Apple Health ecosystem shows us this doesn't have to be hard. In fact, the easier companies make it for us, the more likely we are to be active participants in the process. And the more we participate and the more data we're willing to share (much of it anonymous and aggregated with data from other users), the better the apps will be at making accurate predictions that will make us more likely to use it again. It's a positive health feedback loop—and you're in control.

CHAPTER FOUR:

A PERSONAL TOUR OF YOUR NEW TREATMENT PROTOCOL

"I think it's important to frame that digital health wasn't a stopgap fix for COVID-19, where once the vaccine and return to normal is established, we'll go back. I actually think it's past that. I think we've established providers are able to provide world-class care through these new means." —William Morris, MD, executive medical director of Cleveland Clinic Innovations

The last few chapters have given you a glimpse into the world of doctors, scientists, and innovators who are merging computer science methods with healthcare and biological research. In this chapter and the ones to come, I'll give you a look into what the future could be once these changes take hold.

The Interminable Wait of the Emergency Room

Who among us hasn't taken a trip to the emergency room or urgent care clinic? From weekend warriors who get a little carried away, to sons and daughters who fall on trampolines or get a concussion at the big game, chances are you'll experience the chaos of urgent and emergency healthcare for yourself or a loved one at some point in your life.

The ER experience isn't one that most people would say is good. Overcrowding, long waits, frustrating bureaucratic holdups with insurance or registration, and seemingly arbitrary decisions over who gets seen first. And the cost! At some hospitals, it's bad enough that some patients leave without being seen, only to seek care elsewhere or return later, starting the process all over again. It's no wonder most of us dread the experience—even in the most optimal of situations. Spoiler alert: it doesn't have to be this way.

Decentralized Healthcare: From Hospital to Pharmacy to Home

Imagine you're at your child's soccer practice and he or she collides with another child, both tumbling to the ground. While both kids stand up quickly, your child is holding an arm and complaining that it hurts. It's early on a Saturday morning, and your pediatrician's office is closed. You think your child might need an X-ray and pack up, heading to the ER. Across town, an ambulance is speeding to the hospital with a patient who may have just had a stroke. Already sitting in the ER are twenty-five members of a high school marching band, in town for a competition, but who appear to be suffering from food poisoning from a buffet they ate at the night before. As you're checking in at reception, you ask how long the wait will be and are informed it will be at least three hours. With no urgent care facility in your area and the doctors' offices closed, you have no choice but to wait, trying to find a comfortable chair for you and your child.

In the AI age, when you get sick or need medical attention, your treatment protocol doesn't have to look like this. Your first step, for example, won't be a trip to the doctor's office or hospital, but to a pharmacy or other convenient point-of-care clinic, or even a room in your own home fitted with sensors and connected devices and set up for telehealth. With today's smart TVs and the growing use of smartwatches, connected scales, and blood pressure monitors, it's quite possible that you wouldn't even need additional equipment for a standard appointment. And though emergency care is where this example is centered, these same technologies and procedures could apply for pre- and post-op care, therapy sessions, annual checkups, and so on.

Instead of heading across town to the ER from the soccer field, you take your child home, use your phone to email what happened to your pediatrician, and schedule a ten-minute consult with an online doctor. While you plug in your home portable X-ray machine and scan your insurance card for the telehealth appointment, you get your child settled onto a favorite spot on the couch.

The telehealth visit goes smoothly. The doctor first talks to your child and can see how he or she is holding the arm and how much pain is felt. Next, the doctor guides you through the X-ray process, helping you to precisely position your child's arm for the best image. The machine wirelessly transmits the X-ray to the doctor in a matter of seconds. AI-enabled software helps the doctor read the image quickly, and you are told that the arm isn't broken, it's just bruised. After giving you care instructions, your telehealth visit ends. The time from soccer field collision to receiving a diagnosis—less than thirty minutes. Suddenly, you've got three hours (or more) of your Saturday morning back, your child is already on the way to recovery, and you are relieved of the anxiety over your child's well-being.

While this can sound a little far-fetched, it's not as outlandish as you might think. To be fair, if the child in this example had an obvious fracture or dislocation, needed stitches for a cut, or was in tremendous pain, heading to an urgent care or emergency facility would still be necessary. But for less serious situations, this could be a pretty accurate glimpse into the future.

Multiple companies already manufacture portable X-ray machines meant for specialized situations in home care that can wirelessly transmit data to radiologists for reading. You won't necessarily have to keep medical equipment on hand either. There could be alternatives like public libraries or town facilities that could lend equipment, much the way they lend books, movies, even games and artwork in some areas, or we could see an Uber or Lyft version, where you order the device you need and it is brought to you, sterilized and ready to go, in fifteen minutes or less.

More than a quarter of all emergency visits could be handled at a less-acute facility, like an urgent care office or even the local grocery store. That's partly why it can take someone hours to be seen at an emergency room for a relatively minor complaint, while someone arriving by ambulance for a serious condition is seen more rapidly. Doctors and nurses triage patients—that is, they determine how serious the problem is and decide in what order to see someone based on that assessment.

If you need a physician or specialist, you'll see one virtually—something most of us have become aware of thanks to COVID-19 disruptions. And AI-enabled imaging is already happening. The only things we're missing at the present are X-ray machines that are designed for the average consumer and a platform to seamlessly put it all together. Not far-fetched at all.

Remember that crowded ER with the marching band suffering from presumed food poisoning? Their healthcare experience will also look different in the future. Instead of heading to an ER or an urgent care facility, where they may wait for hours after triage, they'll head directly to the local pharmacy. Even today, CVS and Walgreens are expanding their services beyond simple flu jabs.

If you're unwell, do you really want to have to travel to the doctor for a ten-minute visit (and a twenty-minute wait before you are seen) and still have to pick up a prescription or other wellness aids on the way home? Probably not. CVS, Walgreens, and grocery stores are cutting out the middleman by expanding their in-store health clinics. Today, you can get a school or job physical, receive vaccinations, or see a nurse practitioner or physician assistant for minor health complaints. If you need a prescription, you can walk to the next window and pick it up in minutes. Need some more ibuprofen or bandages too? No problem—they're in Aisle Five. Cough or allergy medicine? Aisle Nine.

The idea of expanding healthcare beyond traditional locations like physicians' offices and hospitals is called decentralization, and it's a strategy that has already worked in other aspects of our lives. You don't need to go to the local bank branch to deposit or withdraw money from your account or to simply check a balance. You can stop by whichever ATM is closest or pull out your phone or laptop. Wherever you are, banking comes to you. For many minor health complaints or injuries, there's little reason we can't do the same in healthcare.

VISION – Health Care Comes to Patients

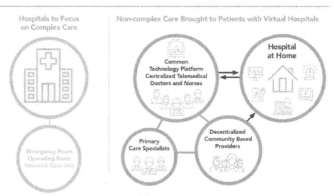

Figure 4.1. Healthcare decentralization.
[https://www.medicallyhome.com/a-virtual-hospital-without-walls/]

Instead of tying up an entire ER for hours while each person is tested for the bacteria making them sick, the marching band director pulls up an app on the phone. Texting with a chatbot or AI-enabled healthcare personal assistant, the director explains the situation. The app has the students head to the nearest pharmacy (GPS directions coming from Google or Apple Maps), where they are tested, prescribed the right medication, and are sent on their way (along with some ginger ale and crackers) in a fraction of the time and at a fraction of the cost. And if patients need something outside the scope of the provider, they can use in-store kiosks or tablets to interact with a remote specialist, who works with the nurse to perform more complex exams or tests. What's more, these apps will be smart—sending patients to nearby pharmacies where the wait in line won't be too long. Just like you can see how long it'll take for a restaurant to see you on a busy Friday night, these apps might show you wait times at a variety of locations and suggest alternatives when it makes sense.

This new continuum of care will decentralize healthcare outside the hospital, which will be primarily reserved for those who are seriously ill or require complex procedures like surgery. So, when the ambulance pulls up to the ER with the patient who may have had a stroke, there won't be a waiting room full of people with more minor complaints, and the rest of the hospital won't be straining under the weight of the countless tests and low-level procedures that could have been done in less acute settings. Instead, the ER will be ready and able, without overwhelming the system, to accommodate the incoming stroke patient, someone with a broken arm or who needs stitches, and more.

The Hospital of the Future

If you do go to the hospital, expect your experience to be AI- and technology-centric. Registration desks will look a lot different. In some hospitals today, they've already been replaced by kiosks where you can scan your license or insurance card and be checked in, automatically sending your insurance information to the billing department or alerting your primary care doctor that you're at the ER. While you can already access some of your electronic health records from your phone, the hospital staff will have them pulled up on their computers, so even when you are away from home, healthcare providers will have access to your health history, the medications you take, and information about the chronic conditions you have or tests you've had done recently.

Though our hypothetical stroke patient, unconscious and arriving to the ER by ambulance, won't necessarily be impressed by the benefits of the AI-enabled hospital of the future, his care and how well he recovers depends on it.

Let's imagine the patient was staying at a hotel by himself. A bystander called the ambulance—or even his Apple Watch—once it determined the man had fallen and wasn't getting up. Paramedics use a secure app on their phone to send an image of the man's driver's license to the hospital. The ER staff uses that to pull up his medical records while he is still en route to the ER, and the system sends an automatic alert to his primary care physician that he's being checked into the ER.

The attending doctor spends the next five minutes scrolling through the patient's medical history, learning that he had been a smoker up to nine months ago, was using a nicotine patch to help him stop smoking, and was taking Prinivil, a medication for high blood pressure. Aside from the high blood pressure, lab tests performed at a routine physical two weeks ago were normal. Before the patient even arrives, the staff has a fairly complete picture of the patient's general health.

Once at the hospital, the real benefits of AI become apparent.

Stroke diagnoses are made by imaging tests, typically by MRIs. But this community hospital doesn't have an expensive MRI machine on site, and the nearest facility that does is more than three hours away—a distance that is too far when every minute after a stroke without treatment could lead to permanent disability. But thanks to AI, this patient can still receive an accurate diagnosis and top care.

Although an MRI scan is out of the question, the hospital does have access to a CT scanner—a faster though less-detailed type of imaging test. Thanks to doctors at hospitals in Boston, there's an AI system that is trained to help radiologists read CT scans of stroke patients. This system, a part of the GE Healthcare Edison Developer Program (you'll hear a lot more about Edison soon), was trained with data from GE MRI and CT scanners in hospitals around the world. Because the machines were built by GE, it gave the engineers and computer scientists easy access to important data for Edison.

Edison scientists used information from patients who received both MRIs and CT scans to "train" the AI to better interpret the lower-resolution CT scans. Doctors could then use CT scans performed in community hospitals to determine which patients could be handled on site and who needed to be stabilized and sent to a more advanced medical center for care. For our hypothetical patient, the news is good: the CT scan indicates that his stroke wasn't severe, and he was admitted to the hospital for treatment.

At this point, you might be thinking there are a few things about this scenario that seem unlikely. For example, if you've ever tried to get a copy of your own medical records, the process is Byzantine and painful. And if a hospital can't afford an MRI machine, how could it possible afford a fancy AI system?

The technology already exists for shared medical records across hospital and healthcare systems. Though not necessarily as complete as the record at your medical home, things like lab results, medications, diagnoses, and allergies can be shared with other hospitals across the nation through health information exchanges or proprietary EHR system platforms. This isn't to say that any doctor anywhere can just look at your health record—that's not the case! Sharing your health record information is limited to situations where it's needed to provide you with medical care. The technology is already being used, and federal standards are leading to increases, year over year, in the number of hospitals and physicians that can share data this way.

AI platforms, like the one I described above that could help a doctor differentiate with lower-resolution imaging which patients need more advanced care, will actually help to level the playing field between community hospitals and academic medical centers. Let's face it, with the growing costs of healthcare, hospitals don't have a blank checkbook—they have to budget and prioritize like the rest of us. If the choice is buying a piece of expensive equipment (to say nothing of the maintenance costs over the expected lifetime of the machine) or investing in an AI platform that helps them maximize their existing equipment and can be updated or improved upon remotely whenever it was needed with minimal maintenance costs, it's not too far of a stretch to imagine the hospital putting the funds toward the more versatile AI platform that can be more easily updated with software releases. And this could have significant positive downstream financial impacts to the patients who get the lower-cost CT imaging with the enhanced AI interpretation.

Decentralized Care with Centralized Monitoring

But what does the hospital of the future really look like? One Canadian hospital already offers patients a glimpse into the future.

Toronto is the capital of the Canadian province of Ontario. Originally three separate community hospitals, the combined Humber River Hospital sits right off the busy Ontario 401 Expressway in the Downsview neighborhood. The sleek beige and glass building opened in 2015 after a four-year construction project, and from the outset it was designed to be innovative.

In 2017, the hospital installed its first AI system, which was designed to track patients as they moved through the hospital. While it might be rare to ever describe an interaction with a hospital as enjoyable or fun, the AI system took aim at one of the more unpleasant sides of hospital crowding—waiting. Imagine never having to wait for a procedure or test past your scheduled appointment time. Or having orderlies ready to move you from one floor to the next at a moment's notice, like they anticipated your next move. Or streamlining the

admissions and discharge processes to be almost …
enjoyable.

For patients, waiting to see the doctor, getting a
test, receiving the right medication, or even leaving for
home when they get better can be more than just
frustrating. Inefficiencies are bad business for hospitals
too. When expensive equipment sits idle, or there aren't
enough beds to fill the need because patients are stuck
waiting in their rooms, or medications expire before they
can be used, it costs hospitals money. But how can
hospitals manage all the patients, staff, equipment, and
facility needs? They need a command center.

In 2017, Humber River Hospital installed exactly
that: a command center full of high-tech screens for video
feeds and patient data. Imagine the deck from the starship
Enterprise brought to life (and down to Earth). From the
command center, staff can monitor everything, from
operating room schedules to how backed up the on-site
laboratory is getting.

Even the building itself is an active participant in
this futuristic hospital. The modern-looking exterior has a
secret—chromatic glass. These special windows
automatically adjust to let in light based on the time of day,
season, or patient preference—all monitored from the
command center. This lets building engineers make the
hospital more energy efficient by controlling heat loss.
Controlling the air conditioning and keeping track of
where people are in the hospital is nice, but this AI system
can do so much more.

The command center is made by GE Healthcare
(the Edison system). In 2019, Humber River Hospital
turned on additional capabilities—"tiles," as the GE
system calls them. The Mother and Baby warning system
is one such module. It monitors both the new baby and the
mom, watching their vital signs for early symptoms of
distress. When an alarm is sounded in the command center,
it also alerts the nursing staff on the unit and provides
information on how to fix the problem.

Edison can also handle imaging data. Humber River recently added a new capability—automatically reading chest X-rays to look for pneumothorax, a kind of collapsed lung. If the system finds an X-ray that it thinks shows a collapsed lung, it alerts the radiologist to review and also lets the patient's care team know. Triaging X-rays in this way can free up valuable time for the radiologists and prioritize cases that are more serious.

The proactive component of the system is what makes the GE Healthcare Edison platform so revolutionary. It's alerting healthcare providers before the patient might be symptomatic by using AI to crunch all the patients' data from connected devices, like automatic blood pressure cuffs or beds that can take temperatures. Triaging patients helps the hospital allocate the right doctor at the right time to the right patient. And Edison can learn by figuring out what data is important—improving the more it is used and the more data it can access for training. Over time, the system will better predict which patients need help and how the doctors should help them, how to best route patients, handle unexpected demands on services (like the surge hospitals saw due to COVID), and keep the hospital clean and comfortable.

While few hospitals have embraced this futuristic platform to the same extent as Humber River, hospitals around the world are using Edison or one if its competitors to rethink how they deliver care and the patient experience. The Cleveland Clinic, for example, is partnering with Luye Medical in Shanghai to build the first Cleveland Clinic Connected project. The medical center, targeted to open in 2024, takes a patient-first approach to hospital design, while advanced technologies, like the kinds I've described, promise to make it one of the most advanced in the world. Closer to home, Boston-area start-up Etiometry is building the visualization platforms and decision support software to enable intensive care doctors anywhere to monitor patients and anticipate a patient's trajectory.

The command center model is one that could go even beyond a bunker-like setting in the hospital. Instead of separating patient care, staff workflows, and facility maintenance, a single command center could serve as the hub on a wheel, sending out directives along the spokes to individual units, like operating rooms or plumbing departments, or specific people, like pipe fitters or a trauma team getting ready for an operation. The benefit of this hub-and-spoke setup is that for situations that impact multiple groups of people or locations in the hospital, the command center works across departments at the same time.

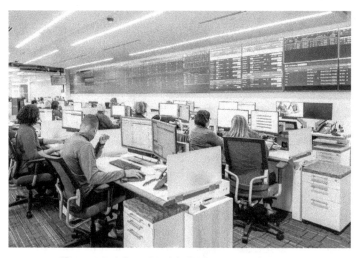

Figure 4.2. AdventHealth (FL) command center.
[https://healthtechmagazine.net/article/2020/02/look-inside-adventhealths-massive-new-command-center]

Today, if the emergency room gets an influx of patients, from a multi-vehicle accident or pandemic, for example, that kind of situation could result in one or more hospitals being placed on a "bypass" status, where ambulances are redirected to other facilities that have open beds and available personnel. If the catastrophe is large enough, that could mean traveling miles away from the site in order to find an open ER.

With the command center model, hospitals can locate and reposition healthcare workers from other areas of the medical center or surrounding physician offices, work with the facilities department to make sure there is adequate seating and equipment in the ER and waiting areas, and reschedule noncritical patients for certain tests or procedures until the surge is over. The result is a hospital that runs more efficiently and provides a better experience for patients.

From *Fortnite* to Facial Reconstruction: How Video Games and AI Are Transforming Surgery

Ever wonder about the training doctors and surgeons undergo? How can they improve on their hand-eye coordination? You might be surprised to learn that research has shown that doctors who play video games perform better than their colleagues who don't at certain skills like laparoscopic surgery, and they make fewer errors on training tasks. The benefit of playing video games doesn't end after medical school or residency, though, and the types of "games" go far beyond *Fortnite*.

Virtual reality for science and medicine has been around for a while. Individuals studying to become doctors have used the technology to practice giving patients stitches, conduct an exam, or perform virtual autopsies. The technology is helping to standardize medical education: every student, no matter where that student is in school, can work on the same "patients" before moving on to the real thing.

If you need something more than just stitches for a cut, AI will improve your chances of success. For example, your surgeon may have already "operated" on you virtually first, using a virtual reality headset or augmented reality, which overlays digital projections onto real-life objects. Surgeons can practice complicated techniques or difficult procedures over and over without risk to the patient. They can even adjust the settings, practicing what to do if a complication arises, or if they find something unexpected once they get started.

Even though virtual reality and AI are making surgeons even better, they might not be the ones performing the operation. Your surgeon might instead oversee it, allowing more precise surgical robots to do the work.

Imagine having your appendix removed while you're physically in Kansas City, and the surgeon is in New York City? Or delicate brain surgery for a tumor while you're in Toledo, but the surgical oncologist is in Cleveland? What about treating a patient with a broken bone who just happens to have COVID or Ebola? Sound impossible?

In 2001, surgeons in New York successfully removed the gall bladder of a sixty-eight-year-old woman living in France without complication. Since then, the field of "telerobotic surgery" has exploded, with platforms called Aesop, Zeus, and da Vinci, names that conjure ideas of strength, knowledge, and innovation. Patients need not worry about being left stranded if the Internet goes down, because on-site medical staff can intervene if needed.

What's more, these long-distance surgical feats can be a solution to the problem of delivering care during a pandemic or outbreak of infectious disease. Not only can the technique help to keep the medical team safe—it can also mean that hospitals can continue to offer care and elective procedures rather than having to cancel everything. Combined with post-procedure telehealth visits, patient care could continue relatively normally.

Sidebar:
Why Robots Will Never Fully Replace Doctors: The Essential Role of Humans in Healthcare

Are you starting to feel a little anxious that instead of a friendly face greeting you when you wake up from surgery, you'll be met with a coldly clinical robot? Fear not—the human side of medicine isn't going away anytime soon. Even in *Star Trek*, human doctors were the ones wielding the tricorder, interpreting the data, and doling out the treatment.

First, there's something to be said that medicine is both an art and a science. Sometimes, to get to the correct diagnosis, doctors need a little bit of the "art" – nonlinear thinking—that AI systems just don't have. Remember that AI systems are basically math sentences put together and depend on the data they're fed. So, if you have a patient that doesn't look like other patients, or a situation that is completely different than anything seen before, the AI system's training probably won't be able to solve the problem—but a really creative doctor might.

Second, though there have been countless articles trying to position the situation in a man vs. machine fight, the reality is that machines and tools like AI are more likely to help doctors and health professionals do their jobs better, more efficiently, and (hopefully) with less stress than today. The inventions of MRIs and CT scanners didn't lead to the end of the X-ray machine—instead, doctors learned to recognize when to use one over the other.

Finally, there are some medical tasks that a human simply has to perform, at least for the long foreseeable future. Can you envision a time when a robot will draw blood, perform the Heimlich maneuver on a choking victim, or deliver a baby? While AI-enabled robots that could technically perform those tasks might be a part of some future many, many years down the road, I have a hard time envisioning any woman in labor that would be OK with robot arms delivering her baby.

So, while an article will come out every few months or so with a doomsday prophecy that AI is going to eliminate doctors and that robots will take over medicine, I think it's safe to say it's not happening. There will be some jobs that humans do today that will be automated, like digitizing paper medical records, dealing with the reams of paperwork, or combing through medical literature. But the literal human touch in medicine can't be duplicated.

—End Sidebar—

Replacement Parts from a 3D Printer

While long-distance robotic surgery can solve the problem of getting the doctors to the patients, what about when the patient needs a new organ, like a kidney? Stories about patients languishing on transplant waiting lists for years, getting sicker all the while, are plentiful. More than one hundred thousand men, women, and children are on the US national transplant waiting list in 2020, and seventeen people die every day while waiting for an organ to become available.

Scientists are starting to use 3D printing to fill this need with cells, tissues, or even whole organs that were made from 3D printing. Nonmedical 3D printing uses resin or other material to precisely create an object. Initially too expensive for home use, many public libraries and schools installed 3D printers for guests and students to try out the devices, creating small tchotchkes like figurines or helping users to better understand geometry with hollow cubes and geodesic shapes. The user programs the device, telling it where to put the resin, adding to the object one tiny layer at a time.

Medical researchers have even used 3D printing to splint broken arms, creating a personalized cast that can be showered in (without wrapping it first in a plastic garbage bag), is more comfortable than the traditional plaster cast, and lets doctors use ultrasound to speed up the healing process. 3D-printed prosthetics are already reality.

The process is obviously more complicated when you're trying to build an ear. To start, the materials used to create the object aren't plastic resins but are cells—the building blocks of tissues or organs. Unlike plastic, cells aren't so forgiving of hostile environments, so researchers have to develop methods to keep the cells alive. There's also the problem of needing different types of cells. If you're trying to make a 3D-printed ear, for example, you'd need hair cells, epithelial cells, and neural cells. Each cell type might have different requirements to keep it alive or need different hormones at precise times to tell the cell what to do. The process becomes even more complicated if you're trying to build a kidney or liver.

If you start with a two-dimensional image, like a picture, there needs to be a way to turn it into a 3D image. Imagine taking a picture of someone head-on and using just that picture to create a bust of that person's head. It would be tough without a way to know just how far the nose stuck out or the chin receded. AI software is used to translate the 2D images into 3D models in a process called segmentation. The better the AI algorithms are at predicting those 3D images, the better the result. Bones and ear tissue made with 3D printers are already in clinical testing, with 3D-printed tissue for the heart, lungs, esophagus, kidneys, liver, ovaries, and muscles currently in development. In another decade, those transplant waiting lists could be a thing of the past.

The Future You: Tomorrow's Patient Today

In this chapter, I've shown you a glimpse into what the future of your healthcare might look like. From checkups at the grocery store and home "office" visits to a whole new kind of hospital that looks more like science fiction than today's reality and growing replacement body parts in a 3D printer, AI is changing where and how you get your care.

The Cleveland Clinic, for one, has embraced decentralized care by partnering with pharmacy giant CVS's in-store MinuteClinics. So when you head to the drugstore for a quick checkup, flu shot, or strep throat test, the results are shared with your regular healthcare team and placed in your electronic health record. If the problem is more than the MinuteClinic's nurse practitioner can handle alone, on-site telehealth visits with Cleveland Clinic specialists are available.

As we saw in Chapter Three, we are doing a lot more these days with our smartphones than simply making phone calls or texting—the devices are practically another member of our healthcare team. There are apps that tell you the most likely cause of your symptoms, and how soon you should contact a doctor, and fitness apps that integrate with health apps that integrate with your electronic health record, giving you (and your healthcare providers) more insight into your overall health and well-being.

Now, imagine combining the hospital command center model with decentralized care. It shouldn't matter where you are—at home, at the store, or in the hospital—if your healthcare team can work together seamlessly to give you the best care possible. It might not matter where the command center is either. Cleveland Clinic is once again a pioneer in this aspect. Doctors remotely monitored noncritically ill patients at Cleveland Clinic and three other regional hospitals from an off-site location and compared their results to how patients did the year before. The researchers determined that the remote monitoring teams identified critical patient issues and alerted on-site care teams sooner than they would have otherwise under the traditional model. Importantly, the remote monitoring didn't have negative consequences for patients.

In the years to come, hospitals will use remote monitoring combined with systems like Edison to proactively protect patients from adverse reactions or complications. Patients living in rural locations or areas without access to certain specialists will use telehealth and supervised robotic surgeries to expand their access to both primary healthcare as well as distant specialists. And we'll be able to meet the global organ shortage to reduce the length of time it takes someone to get a transplant.

Are You Ready for the Future?

Why should you care about decentralized healthcare, AI command centers, and doctors who play *Fortnite* or *Among Us*? While not everyone has access to a Humber River Hospital, with its fancy windows or hub-and-spoke model, AI is being integrated everywhere, giving you, the patient, faster, better care wherever you live.

What you can do now:
- Download an app that can help you identify the cause of your symptoms—and tell you when you should seek professional care urgently, or if you can safely hold off until your doctor's office opens in the morning. There are already apps that are aimed at helping doctors puzzle out difficult diagnoses, such as Isabel or DynaMed, but fewer options for patients, like Ada. Still, your healthcare provider might have some suggestions for you, and this is an area of interest. Expect to see new apps for this in the upcoming years.
- Learn if visits to the doctor or hospital for minor illnesses, tests, physicals, or minor procedures can be done via telehealth, at a retail clinic, or urgent care. You might find that it could save you time and money. Some hospitals, healthcare systems, and insurance companies are even creating their own apps for this purpose—so your doctor might already be able to recommend one to you.
- Have access to a 3D printer and want to help those who need prosthetics? There are numerous online communities and schematics that can be used to create low-tech prosthetics for those in need. Look on social media platforms to get involved.

- Be flexible and adaptable (as much as you can). The technologies described in this chapter, and throughout this book, are evolving so rapidly that it can be difficult to keep up. Start-ups emerge on the scene only to quietly exit a short time later. Features of apps you love might change, leaving you missing a key function while giving you others.

CHAPTER FIVE:

UNLOCKING THE LANGUAGE OF LIFE

"The human genome is a life written in a book where every word has been written before. A story endlessly rehearsed." —*Johnny Rich, author of* The Human Script

In 2006, a small start-up in California launched with the mission to help people understand and benefit from their genetics. It was a worthy goal, coming only three years after the official end of the Human Genome Project. The tech-savvy cofounders promised to make learning about genetics easy and fun. Spit-kit events were profiled in *The New York Times* alongside society cocktail parties, and participants could find out if they had genetic markers for red hair, the ability to smell asparagus in urine, or ancient Neanderthal DNA. That start-up, 23andMe, has risen to become the internationally recognized leader in the marketing of genetic tests directly to consumers—and virtually a household name, with more than twelve million customers, FDA-approved tests, and agreements with pharmaceutical companies for things like cancer treatments.

To understand why this is so groundbreaking, let's take a step back to the mid-1960s. At that time, scientists knew that DNA was the genetic building block of life, that there were twenty-three pairs of chromosomes in humans, and James Watson, Francis Crick, and Maurice Wilkins had been awarded the Nobel Prize in Physiology or Medicine for their discovery of the structure of DNA. One scientist estimated there were more than 6.5 million genes, or protein-coding sequences of DNA, while others gave ranges from fifty thousand to more than one hundred forty thousand. Even the experts were all over the place in their estimates, all based on science and math, but none fully grasping the details we now know today. As time went on, more of the secrets of the human genome were uncovered.

Fast-forward another thirty years to the time when I was working for Applied Biosystems Inc., a company that would become one of the names synonymous with Human Genome Project technology. By then, the estimated number of genes had been scaled back to around one hundred thousand. Some genes were already known to cause certain diseases, and we were on track to developing the initial drafts of the human genome. By the time the Human Genome Project came to a close in 2003, the estimated number of genes had dropped to around thirty thousand, and we were edging ever closer to utter transformation of medicine and health research.

Sidebar:
Molecular Genetics in a Nutshell

What is a gene? What is DNA? Just how many chromosomes do we have? Why does this even matter?

The human genome is the language of life, a code or blueprint containing three billion different letters of DNA that spell out what makes you human and uniquely you. Molecular genetics is the method we use to understand that language of life.

Let's start with the basics. Deoxyribonucleic acid, or DNA for short, is the building block of the human genome. It's made of chemicals, called nucleotide bases, that are joined in long chains and paired with an opposite strand, creating a double helix. This double helix is probably what you envision when someone mentions DNA (Figure 5.1). The nucleotide bases pair with each other in a specific way, but along the strand itself, the order of the bases differs slightly. Guanine (G) always pairs with cytosine (C) and adenine (A) pairs with thymine (T), but between people, on one strand the order might be GAC while another person's strand in the same place would have GAG or even TCA.

These long sequences of nucleotides are broken up into smaller packages of different lengths called chromosomes. Humans have forty-six chromosomes (twenty-three pairs). The number of chromosomes varies by organism: dogs have seventy-eight chromosomes and bananas have thirty-three! Scientists have learned that how complicated an animal or plant is doesn't really have bearing on the number of chromosomes it has.

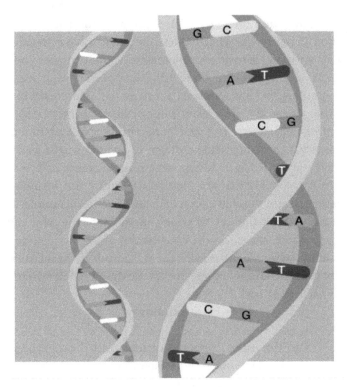

Figure 5.1. The DNA double helix.
[https://www.genome.gov/About-Genomics/Introduction-to-Genomics]

Genes are specific sequences of DNA that tell the cellular machinery to make a specific protein—scientists call them "protein coding regions." We now know that there are less than twenty thousand genes in the human genome—a far cry from those early estimates of more than one hundred thousand! There are also regulatory regions of DNA that determine when a gene might get translated into a protein or how much of a protein to make.

In general, from person to person along nearly six billion places (three billion on each strand or "side" of the DNA helix), the order of each strand is 99.9 percent identical. Those similarities, the blueprints, are what make humans ... well ... humans instead of turtles or birds or apples. But the remaining 0.01 percent of the roughly six million variants are what makes one person have freckles while another remains unblemished, what makes one person have curly hair while another doesn't, what leads one person to develop breast cancer or diabetes while another doesn't. One variant might cause a protein called a tumor suppressor to stop being produced, and cancer might start to grow, while a different variant might lead a growth factor to shut down—stopping a cancer cell. Not all of these variants are detrimental to your health—whether or not you have attached earlobes, for example. If you can unlock the key to your genetic language, you can start to crack the code on your health and who you are, including what might make you sick, how to prevent or delay disease, and whether you are destined to be an early riser or a night owl.

—End Sidebar—

By the time Anne Wojcicki and her partners founded 23andMe, our understanding of the human genome had grown exponentially. We were closing in on new gene discoveries at a rapid-fire pace, and the number of labs offering genetic testing had begun to flourish. Researchers were beginning to draw correlations between specific genetic variants—those tiny differences in our DNA—and diseases and traits using a technique called genome-wide association studies (GWAS). In a GWAS, scientists compared the genomes of people with and without a trait, such as whether you thought cilantro tasted like soap, by comparing their DNA at hundreds of thousands of different places in the genome. The early

23andMe Personal Genome Service used published GWAS to give customers a look at how their genetic variants impacted their risk of having or developing dozens of disorders and non-disease traits.

Nearly twenty years after the first drafts of the human genome were published in *Science* and *Nature* journals, having your whole genome sequenced costs less than $1,000 and can be done in a few hours—not the thirteen-year, $3 billion effort it took to sequence the first human genome. Even more impressive? That cost continues to drop: in 2020, Chinese scientists announced they had sequenced the human genome for a mere $100! While the technological breakthroughs are nothing short of extraordinary, the far-reaching health impacts of the Human Genome Project surpass them. In this chapter, I'll describe three ways why unlocking the secrets of your genome matters to your health now and how the "future you" might not be written in DNA stone.

Pharmacogenomics: Preventing Bad Drug Reactions

It's long been known that there are many factors that determine a patient's response to a particular drug, like the dose and what other medications they might be taking. Even in the early 1900s, doctors were aware that some patients would respond differently to medications. English physician Sir Archibald Garrod, who discovered the rare metabolic disease alkaptonuria (aka "black urine disease"), wrote in 1908:

> *"Every active drug is a poison, when taken in large enough doses; and in some subjects a dose which is innocuous to the majority of people has toxic effects, whereas others show exceptional tolerance of the same drug."*

We now know a lot more about the role that genetics plays in disease and have begun to tease out the differences in drug response documented by Dr. Garrod more than a century ago. Pharmacogenomics is the study of how genes affect the response to drugs. It is the cornerstone of personalized (or precision) medicine.

In general, a person with a specific diagnosis, say high cholesterol, will be treated like most other patients with the same diagnosis. A doctor might prescribe a medication, and if the patient responds favorably, the patient will continue the treatment. If the patient has a negative reaction to the drug or fails to respond—let's say the high cholesterol stays the same instead of decreasing— the doctor would then make a change to the prescription, trying another.

For some conditions, like depression, there may be more than a dozen different medications that could be prescribed, and the patient might have to try more than a handful before landing on the right one. Every time a new medication is tested, the patient has to wait a certain period of time to know whether or not it is working, all along hoping not to have one of the countless side effects that appear in tiny type at the bottom of any drug advertisement. It's basic trial and error; the problem is you are the guinea pig that is being tested. This made sense in the past, since you can only use the tools available to you, but today we can do so much more.

The field of pharmacogenomics offers a better strategy. Instead of treating all patients with the same disorder with the same medication plan, doctors can use genetics to determine which patients are likely to be nonresponders to a drug or figure out who is likely to have a bad side effect and need a different drug (Figure 5.2).

There are now more than one hundred drugs that carry FDA warning labels (called "black box warnings") either requiring genetic testing before the drug is prescribed or where genetic testing is recommended. The conditions these drugs treat range widely from cancer to cystic fibrosis and impact millions of patients every year.

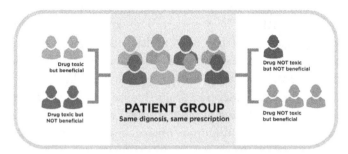

Figure 5.2. Pharmacogenomics Strategy
[Adapted from:
https://www.questdiagnostics.com/home/physicians/testing-services/condition/genetics/pharmacogenomics/]

Now to be clear—not every available medication has a corresponding genetic test, and doctors and hospitals are just starting to make pharmacogenomics testing routinely available. Vanderbilt University Medical Center, in Nashville, Tennessee, was one of the early pioneers in pharmacogenomics. In 2010, Vanderbilt launched Pharmacogenomic Resource for Enhanced Decisions in Care and Treatment (PREDICT) to preemptively test patients who may be at high risk to need specific medications, like statin therapy for high cholesterol, within the next five years. The idea was to test the patients before they started taking the drug—so that the right medication (or dose) could be prescribed the first time around.

A 2014 study found between 91–96 percent of the first ten thousand patients in PREDICT were positive for one or more actionable genetic variants—meaning they would be recommended for a different drug dose or alternate medication entirely. Compare that to today's trial-and-error method of prescribing, where some patients will suffer from serious side effects that make them stop taking the medication or have to switch medications multiple times, and you can understand how getting the right drug to the patient the first time is such a game-changer.

Like most genetic tests, a pharmacogenomic test only needs to be performed once, ideally before the patient has a need for the medication, as modeled by the Vanderbilt PREDICT program. This kind of testing has generally been available only at large academic medical centers under research studies focused on high-risk patients. But now we're seeing a shift in policy. Today, patients who are prescribed drugs that require a genetic test before use and for many drugs where a test is recommended can undergo pharmacogenomics testing, helped in part by the dropping costs of genetic testing. The utility of this strategy is obvious: it prevents adverse drug events and can lead to better patient response to treatment. More importantly, it underscores the benefit of knowing what your DNA says about you.

The Revolutionary Impact of Genetics on Cancer Treatment

Though a cancer diagnosis is never good, today's patients are likely to live longer and have a better quality of life than patients decades ago. A large part of this comes from advancements in genetic testing that help doctors select the best medication for the patient (pharmacogenomics). But others benefit from learning their cancer is part of a hereditary cancer syndrome, and they can take advantage of enhanced screening or preventive treatments.

Patients with breast cancer, for example, can undergo testing to learn if they have a DNA mutation in their genes, a so-called germline mutation, that puts them at risk for developing ovarian cancer as well. *BRCA1* and *BRCA2* are two genes with variants that cause this type of heritable cancer. If a woman with breast cancer has a mutation in one of those genes, she may decide to undergo a surgery to remove her ovaries, since she would be at significantly higher risk of developing ovarian cancer, which is notoriously difficult to diagnose at an early stage.

These types of mutations are part of the individual's genes and are hereditary in nature. For this reason, patients can also learn if they have passed the mutation on to their children, or if other relatives, like a sister, aunt, or parent, also have the mutation, through a process called cascade screening, where at-risk relatives undergo genetic testing to see if they also carry the same mutation as the patient.

But germline testing isn't the only kind of genomic test that cancer patients can benefit from. Cancer tumors that develop in the body can also have their own genetic profile and can be candidates for genetic testing. Mutations found in tumors are called somatic; they are different from germline mutations in that they aren't present in every cell of the body—they arise sometime later in life. Even within a single tumor, the mutations might differ from cell to cell. This is important, because some cancers might respond differently to treatment.

Tumor testing has become tremendously important to cancer care over the last decade as a result of new medications that target specific mutations. What's more, some of these medications are location-agnostic, meaning the site of the tumor isn't the factor driving the choice of medication, it's the specific mutation the tumor has. A groundbreaking clinical trial of patients with twelve different tumor types found that patients with a mutation referred to as deficient mismatch repair (dMMR)/microsatellite instability-high (MSI-H) were sensitive to the treatment pembrolizumab (Keytruda), which has since become the standard of care treatment for patients with these mutations.

As remarkable as all this is, one of the most exciting breakthroughs in cancer care genomics is liquid biopsy. To understand why liquid biopsy is so revolutionary, it helps to compare it to the standard cancer biopsy process.

Liquid Biopsy: The Secrets in Your Blood

Until recently (and still, for most patients), a biopsy, which is a procedure to collect a small part of the tumor (or other sample), is needed to confirm a presumed cancer diagnosis. The patient might head to the doctor because of some worrisome symptoms, get some lab work drawn, wait a week or two for the results, and maybe have an ultrasound, MRI, or other scan. When the results of those studies are complete, the patient returns, perhaps to hear the doctor say that the labs or scan suggest there could be a tumor, and the patient is referred to an oncologist. The next step is often a biopsy to confirm the presumed diagnosis.

In a biopsy, a hollow needle is used to collect some of the cells of the tumor. An ultrasound or CT scan might be used to help guide the placement of the needle, drawing doctors precisely to the tumor location. Multiple biopsies might have to be performed, such as testing lymph nodes or adjacent areas to the suspected tumor, in order to better gauge the extent of the spread of the cancer. Minor pain and discomfort after the biopsy are common. The cells drawn up in the needle are examined by a pathologist to determine whether or not they are cancerous. Other tests that are performed help to identify the specific type of cancer and markers the tumor cells have that could point doctors to the best medication or help determine the overall prognosis (the likely course the patient's disease will take).

Even though biopsy is the gold standard, it's not hard to imagine a few downsides to this process. The needles used to collect the cells are generally larger in diameter than needles used to give a vaccination, for example. But even the largest of needles used for biopsies are relatively small, so it's possible the biopsy will miss the tumor cells and sample normal cells next to the tumor— which is why multiple sites are usually tested. Depending on the location of the tumor, it could be very difficult to reach the tumor without having to go through other tissues or organs. If the tumor is, in fact, cancerous, a few cells from the tumor might be spread to these otherwise healthy tissues during the biopsy when the needle is removed. Though some level of discomfort is expected, some types of biopsy, like bone marrow aspiration, can be painful, even with anesthesia. Lastly, for some cancers, repeated biopsies are needed throughout the course of treatment and follow-up.

Liquid biopsy is an alternative growing in both popularity as well as utility. In liquid biopsy, the patient undergoes a standard blood draw, just like any other lab, such as measuring cholesterol levels or a standard blood count. Sounds incredible, right?

Liquid biopsy works because tumor cells, unlike those of healthy tissues or organs, generally don't hold together particularly well. These cells can break apart from the tumor and then circulate in bodily fluids like blood or urine. The cells themselves might also break up, and their contents, including mutated DNA and biomarkers, can also travel throughout the body. The blood draw captures some of these tumor cells and their cell-free DNA, which is then analyzed in the lab. Importantly, the accuracy of these liquid biopsy tests is generally high.

For cancers that require repeated biopsies to track the progress of treatment or to determine if a cancer in remission is now in recurrence, the ability to swap a relatively painless and fast blood draw for time-consuming, potentially painful biopsies is incredible. And the applications of liquid biopsy continue to expand.

Pancreatic cancer is one of the most common cancers, and the incidence is rising every year. It's estimated that more than fifty-seven thousand new pancreatic cancer cases will be diagnosed, and forty-seven thousand people will die from pancreatic cancer in 2020. The overall prognosis of patients with pancreatic cancer is poor: data from the National Cancer Institute's Surveillance, Epidemiology, and End Results Program from 2010-2016 found a five-year relative survival rate of only 10 percent, but this rate increases to about 20 percent when the cancer can be identified earlier and surgically removed.

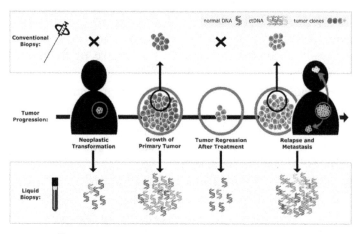

Figure 5.3. Liquid biopsy vs. standard tissue biopsy.
[https://www.genengnews.com/uncategorized/gen-roundup-liquid-biopsies-remain-wait-and-see-for-some-clinicians/]

This is a subject I happen to know quite a bit about, as my mother was diagnosed with pancreatic cancer in early 2012. At the time, liquid biopsy wasn't even a thing, and even genetic testing, something that is pretty much the standard of care for patients with a cancer diagnosis, was only starting to be performed—and only at a few medical centers across the country.

Unfortunately, because there are few symptoms of pancreatic cancer in the early stages of disease, most patients are diagnosed at a late stage, when surgery or chemotherapy may be less effective or no longer an option. A standard pancreatic biopsy has variable accuracy: a false-negative or inconclusive biopsy result is common, so a biopsy method that reduces this variability, improves accuracy, and could be used to diagnose pancreatic cancer at an earlier, more treatable stage, is clearly needed.

One recent clinical trial found that liquid biopsy could diagnose patients with pancreatic tumors eligible for surgery, and another study found it could confirm detection of eight different cancer types, demonstrating its utility for this purpose. Doctors and scientists are working on applying liquid biopsy for prostate cancer, pediatric brain tumors, and more. Moving beyond the simple blood draw, there is interest in using liquid biopsy to monitor more than just cancer cells. New cancer treatments, called immunotherapies, attempt to harness the patient's immune system to go after the cancer. Liquid biopsy could be used to monitor the immune response, letting doctors know easily and quickly when treatment stops working.

The benefits of liquid biopsy have been proven already for many patients, and its use is expected to increase as the technology matures. But why not take this technology and turn it on healthy people, monitoring them yearly for cancer before any symptoms even arise?

What sounds like science fiction is moving closer to reality. In April 2020, a team of scientists from Johns Hopkins University and Geisinger Health System presented findings from a preliminary study that does just that. In the study, more than ten thousand healthy women had blood taken from them and analyzed with a liquid biopsy approach, where researchers scanned their blood for cancer markers. A team of physicians looked to see if there was a noncancer reason for any positive result—remember, these were healthy patients with no prior evidence of cancer. If no other reason could be the cause of the finding, the patients received additional screening and were followed for a year to see if they were diagnosed with cancer. The researchers determined that the liquid biopsy test was able to detect more than 50 percent of cancers, more than double the number found by traditional screenings, and 65 percent of these were early stage (local or regional tumors).

Liquid biopsy tests are bringing us closer to a pan-cancer blood test. A test that could be done as routinely for cancer as getting your cholesterol or blood pressure checked are for heart disease. A test that could find cancer at its earliest stages, when treatments are less invasive, and the prognosis is best. A simple blood test, instead of a painful biopsy, to let us know when the treatment stops working and to direct doctors toward the best medication. It's the epitome of personalized medicine and finally within reach—possible only by unlocking the DNA secrets in our blood.

Sequenced at Birth: How DNA Sequencing Is Transforming Pregnancy and Beyond

Have you ever seen "PHENYLKETONURICS: CONTAINS PHENYLALANINE" on a can of Diet Coke or on a pack of chewing gum and wondered what that was about? These labels have everything to do with newborn screening and an inherited metabolic disease.

Few times in a person's life are filled with greater joy (or greater anxiety) than pregnancy. Over the course of nine months, everything from pink vs. blue, which diapers to use, pacifier or not, is agonized over. For some parents, the questions move far beyond infancy to preschool waiting lists or in which school district to purchase a home. The questions and advice from well-meaning family and friends seem endless.

One of the biggest unknowns expectant parents face is whether the child will be healthy. For most, this question is basically rhetorical. Without a family history of an inherited illness, the general expectation is that the new baby will be perfect. For some families, the waiting period between the positive pregnancy test and counting the newborn's fingers and toes is excruciatingly long. But checking over a newborn doesn't end there.

You might be aware that soon after a baby is born, their heel is pricked, and the blood collected for state-mandated newborn screening programs. These programs test the newborn for a variety of conditions, from hearing loss to metabolic disorders. Many of these are treatable when caught early, so testing newborns could have a dramatic impact on their lives.

State and national newborn screening programs got their starts in the 1960s, when Dr. Robert Guthrie developed a test for phenylketonuria (PKU). PKU is a metabolic disease caused by an enzyme deficiency. This deficiency prevents the body from processing a part of a protein, phenylalanine, which builds up in the person's body and causes brain damage. If diagnosed quickly, soon after birth, treatment can prevent brain damage.

Approximately one in ten thousand babies have PKU, but the symptoms don't begin to show up immediately. Unfortunately, the brain damage is irreversible. Strict adherence to a low-phenylalanine diet can prevent the intellectual disability that results from the high levels of phenylalanine. (This is why diet soda and other foods containing phenylalanine have that warning on their labels.) Dr. Guthrie's test proved to be more accurate than a urine-based test, and he became a crusader for testing all newborns before they even left the hospital.

Fast-forward more than half a century, and newborn screening can identify dozens of disorders. Though newborn screening panels are specific to each state, there are a core number of diseases and conditions all states test for. But these discrepancies between states mean that babies born in California will be screened for sixty-four conditions, those in Kansas for thirty-two, and newborns in Florida for fifty-six. The number of disorders tested for is partly a consequence of the state's population and the overall prevalence of that condition in the state. But these state-by-state differences in newborn screening panels mean that some disorders are still missed. When the timing of the diagnosis can mean the difference between a symptom-free life and one with serious disability, thousands of families are at risk.

There is a lot of interest, therefore, in using genetic sequencing as a complement to newborn screening. While not every metabolic disorder or other condition can be identified through genetic testing, newborn genomic sequencing could greatly expand the number of conditions tested, lead to earlier treatment and intervention for some diseases, and help level the playing field for families across the country.

The BabySeq Project is an attempt to do just that. In 2017, doctors at Brigham and Women's Hospital and Boston Children's Hospital published a paper outlining the randomized controlled trial of genetic counseling and sequencing in both healthy and critically ill newborns in the intensive care unit (ICU). Because genomic sequencing has the potential to uncover mutations that might not be relevant for decades, the doctors grouped results into three main categories, encompassing about one thousand genes.

First, they reported results with high predictive value; that is, the genomic mutations were highly predictive for a disorder. This category included disorders where a rapid diagnosis would prevent a diagnostic odyssey for the patient and their family—something that often occurs when the child has symptoms that overlap many different disorders or have rarely been seen before. Other disorders in this category may have treatment options, or diseases that present later in childhood, but where early intervention can make a difference. PKU, mentioned earlier, is also in this group. The last group of disorders in this category includes those where there is no current treatment, but having the diagnosis can be beneficial for the family for future family planning or could improve the quality of life of the person with options like comfort care. Diseases in this subgroup include Rett syndrome, a disease that affects girls ages six-to-eighteen months and is characterized by change in development, intellectual disability, scoliosis, and loss of social interaction. While Rett syndrome is not curable, treatments are directed at improving quality of life, like physical therapy to help with hand problems or aid with feeding and diapering.

The second group of results included disorders with either a childhood or adolescent onset where early intervention or treatment could improve the long-term outcomes for the patient. Some inherited cancer syndromes fall into this category, because the patient could undergo cancer screening before symptoms develop or at an earlier age than is normally recommended. Inherited heart conditions, such as cardiomyopathies, are also included in this group. In addition to genes that fit in these categories, the BabySeq study team later added a small number of genes responsible for adult-onset disorders—results that could have a dramatic impact on families who were found to have a mutation.

The third category of results were ones the doctors excluded from reporting. You might wonder why doctors would choose not to provide information related to a disease or condition. The answer is complicated. For some results in this category, even if the genomic mutation was highly heritable, there might not be any evidence today that screening for this in childhood leads to early detection or dramatically improves the overall outcome for the patient. For others in this category, the mutation might have what scientists call "low penetrance"—even if a person has the mutation, there's no guarantee that they will develop the disorder. A mutation in the *FS* gene that can lead to an increased risk of deep vein thrombosis (DVT) is one example—you could have the mutation but never develop a DVT throughout your entire life! For others, there may not be enough evidence right now linking the disease with the mutation.

BabySeq has had a dramatic impact on several families' lives already.

Cora Stetson is one of the 159 babies in the BabySeq Project with a result that had an immediate and lasting impact on her health and well-being. Cora was found to have a mutation in a gene that leads to biotin deficiency, a vitamin important for hearing, vision, and even seizures and behavioral disorders. Thankfully, the treatment is fairly simple: a daily dose of the vitamin. Now an active and healthy preschooler, Cora's biotin deficiency is treated with a simple dose of the vitamin in her morning yogurt, and her family credits the BabySeq Project and its doctors for their positive outcome.

It's not just the babies who are benefiting from BabySeq. A few years ago, parents of a healthy newborn were approached by study personnel to see if they would be interested in participating. The family thought, "Why not?" With their family history being fairly benign and absent of serious conditions, they weren't anticipating much coming from the genetic test and counseling but imagined a positive test for their son might have implications when he reached adulthood.

A few months later, the couple were shocked to receive a call from BabySeq staff letting them know their son had a *BRCA* mutation—a mutation associated with the development of hereditary breast and ovarian cancer in adulthood. For men, this means not only an increased risk of developing breast cancer, but also prostate cancer (men don't have ovaries, so they aren't at risk of ovarian cancer). However, the results would have practically no impact until their son, by then just a few months old, would reach adulthood, when he would be eligible for increased screening.

While this was unexpected and a lot to take in, the news didn't stop there. The scientists had figured out which parent had passed on the mutation to their newborn—meaning *they* would also be at risk of developing cancer. And unlike for their son, this information was actionable—now.

The baby's mother (I'll call her Sarah; she wishes to remain anonymous at this time) said that the news spurred a whirlwind of activity. Although the BabySeq study had found the mutation in her sample as well, she needed to undergo formal genetic counseling and clinical testing to confirm the research result. She sees an oncologist to help her make sense of her risks for breast and ovarian cancer in the future and gets either a mammogram or an MRI every six months to monitor for signs of early breast cancer, and a pelvic ultrasound and special bloodwork to look for signs of ovarian cancer. In the future, Sarah says that she'll undergo both a double mastectomy and an oophorectomy (removal of the ovaries).

I asked Sarah about her family history. She said that the result made her take a closer look at her family history. She discovered that two uncles have prostate cancer and her aunt had a double mastectomy for breast cancer. Sharing this information with family has been complicated. "I started with my aunts, not my cousins directly," Sarah said, to see if they wanted to make any health decisions around this.

When I asked Sarah if she or her husband had any regrets about participating in the program, she replied, "I don't regret it, but it has been an emotional ride that I had not expected when we, off the cuff, said 'yes' in a hospital room four years ago." She views having the additional information as beneficial overall and is glad to share her story if it helps someone else.

Project Baby Bear, at San Diego's Rady Children's Institute for Genomic Medicine, is using rapid genome sequencing to help diagnose newborns and babies in regional NICUs and pediatric ICUs (PICUs). What makes Baby Bear and similar programs unique, compared to standard genomic testing, is that they can turn around results in a few days instead of the current multiple weeks or months. For critically ill babies, this timing can truly mean the difference between life and death, and can help parents and doctors make rapid decisions about medications and procedures that could have taken months without sequencing.

Along the way, the BabySeq Project, Project Baby Bear, and others that are part of the National Institutes of Health's Newborn Sequencing in Genomic Medicine and Public Health (NSIGHT) studies, are helping doctors and researchers grapple with technical challenges (how quickly can you get results back to doctors and how often should you reanalyze genomic sequencing results) and thorny ethical conundrums (will parents refuse some care if their newborn is found to have an incurable disease?). What parents of newborns think as valuable information may not be the same as what the scientists think. And the costs of genomic sequencing, while definitely dropping and a tiny fraction of the cost it once took to sequence the human genome, are still a lot higher than newborn screening using the traditional methods. The costs to analyze that data, or reanalyze it at some point in the future when new discoveries could be made, are another factor.

Despite the ongoing debates and challenges, it's hard to argue that newborn genomic screening isn't yet ready for prime time—for some patients. Project Baby Bear led to substantial lower healthcare costs ($2.5 million!) in large part because doctors were able to give the sick babies the right treatment more quickly and reduce the length of hospital stays and number of additional tests, like invasive scopes or spinal taps, that would have been needed in the past to reach a diagnosis. Children's Mercy Kansas City proved rapid whole genome sequencing in the NICU/PICU helped doctors to make patient management decisions, and more than a quarter of the families had genetic counseling following results. Long-term follow-up of patients enrolled in the NSIGHT studies will help to quantify the impact on healthcare utilization (the number and cost of additional procedures, screenings, referrals, etc.) and downstream family consequences: Are current or future siblings at risk for an inherited condition? Did the sequencing help the family make an early education plan for the child?

This last point isn't one to overlook. When a newborn baby or child receives a genetic diagnosis, the family can feel isolated, anxious, and at a loss for what to do next. Genetic counseling is an essential component of genome medicine, helping families to better understand who in the family is also at risk, and working in concert with physicians to coordinate care. While the child's medical care might be planned, social media is helping families connect with others for social and emotional support in caring for a special-needs child.

The question remains whether newborn genomic sequencing is the right test for healthy newborns. Results from the BabySeq Project highlight some of the challenges. First, genomic sequencing can't replace some of the standard newborn screening tests that are universally performed (though as I mentioned previously, the content of these screening tests varies widely). Second, the cost of genomic sequencing can't be ignored—they are still substantial today, though the costs continue to drop. For sick babies, the financial benefits can be readily seen, like at Rady Children's, but for healthy babies, it's far more complicated and may not actually result in cost savings over the course of a lifetime, if you factor in additional screening or procedures for a disease they aren't guaranteed to even get. Then, you have to consider the impacts to the families. For such a new technology, there just isn't a lot of data to rely on. Still, newborn genomic sequencing is steadily expanding across the country and around the world—saving newborns' lives and helping their families plan for the future.

The Future You: Rewriting the Language of Life

So far, we've seen how unlocking the secrets hidden in your DNA can help you get the right drug the first time, preventing potentially catastrophic side effects from the wrong medication dose or drug; how liquid biopsy is changing cancer surveillance and helping to end painful tumor biopsies; and how DNA sequencing is reshaping baby's first test. This next section will show you how scientists are taking things one step further to rewrite the language of life.

Sickle cell anemia and beta thalassemia are two blood disorders. In patients with sickle cell disease, red blood cells, the normally round cells that carry oxygen through the body, are misshapen into crescent, or sickle, shape. The sickle shape prevents the red blood cells from smoothly traveling through the body's blood vessels and sometimes cause clots as they bunch up. This is extremely painful and can even lead to strokes and death. Patients with beta thalassemia have low levels of hemoglobin, a protein that binds to oxygen in red blood cells for transport around the body. The result is a shortage of red blood cells, called anemia, which can cause extreme tiredness, weakness, or put patients at risk of developing blood clots.

What do these two blood diseases have in common? They are both caused by mutations in the *HBB* gene.

Sidebar:
What Is Gene Editing with CRISPR?

Imagine your DNA is stretched out before you like the thread in the hem of your shirt. A mutation in the DNA would be like a snag in the thread halfway around the hem. You need to fix it, but the rest of the hem is fine. Wouldn't it be great to just snip out the offending snag with a tiny pair of scissors and replace it with a new thread? Now imagine doing just that to actual DNA sequences. In people. This is exactly what gene editing with CRISPR, an acronym for "clustered regularly interspaced short palindromic repeats," attempts to do (Figure 5.4). It's like a Swiss Army knife for DNA mutations.

So what is CRISPR, exactly, and how does it work?

Our DNA is packaged into chromosomes, just like other animals and plants. Genes, the sections of our DNA that are responsible for creating proteins, aren't unique to humans. It might seem a little weird that a banana tree might have a gene that humans have, but so do cats, dogs, and hummingbirds. For example, of the roughly twenty thousand human genes, nearly sixteen thousand have a comparable gene in domestic cats. The functions of the genes are pretty similar from species to species, which lets scientists study a particular genetic mutation in an animal model, say fruit flies, instead of people. And when they discover how something works in an animal or bacteria or yeast, it could have implications in humans too.

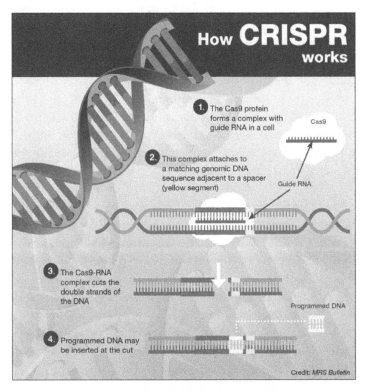

Figure 5.4. What is CRISPR?
[https://www.cambridge.org/core/journals/mrs-bulletin/news/crispr-implications-for-materials-science]

For a while, scientists knew that there were sections of DNA in bacteria that repeated and thought they might have something to do with how bacteria fend off viruses (Yes—even bacteria can be infected with viruses!). They called these repetitive, short segments "clustered regularly interspaced short palindromic repeats," or

CRISPR. Some of these CRISPRs exactly match viral sequences. When a virus invades a bacterial cell, the bacterial DNA machinery gets to work and transcribes the DNA sequence into RNA. That RNA helps the bacteria protect itself by bringing a special protein called a nuclease (Cas) over to the viral DNA to cut it up. So, if bacteria were to "catch a cold," this is how they could deal with it. But these CRISPR aren't only found in bacteria—they're also found in humans.

Researchers wondered if they could make a CRISPR that would work with the nuclease, the CRISPR/Cas, to cut the genome in a very specific place and no other, such as where there was a mutation. Once the genome was cut at the location the scientists wanted, they could insert a new sequence in that place or use the cell's own machinery to rebuild the DNA sequence correctly. It worked.

In 2020, a pair of scientists, American Jennifer Doudna and Emmanuelle Charpentier from France, shared the Nobel Prize in Chemistry for their discoveries of the CRISPR/Cas system. Part of what makes the CRISPR discovery so astounding is that it can be applied to animals and plants. Imagine curing hereditary cancers or other diseases in humans. Creating a new crop of plants that's always resistant to pests, blights, poor soils, or needs less water. Breeding heartier and healthier livestock. That's some Swiss Army knife. ☺

—End Sidebar—

In early July 2019, Victoria Gray, a Mississippi woman with debilitating sickle cell disease, underwent a procedure with CRISPR. During this procedure, her bone marrow was removed and CRISPR used to carefully edit the *HBB* mutation, so her cells would instead produce a working form of hemoglobin instead of the mutated version, before putting the bone marrow back. The doctors' expectations were that the cells producing the working form of hemoglobin would compensate for the mutated version her cells were producing. If enough of her cells produced the new version, it could spare the patient the excruciating bouts of pain she suffered and stop further damage to her heart from sickle cell disease.

GENE EDITING WITH CRISPR

CRISPR-Cas9 gene editing is helping to tackle sickle-cell disease in two ways.

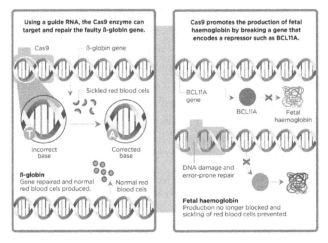

Figure. 5.5. How CRISPR fixes sickle cell disease.
[Adapted From: https://www.nature.com/articles/549S28a]

A year later, the patient and her medical team are cautiously calling the revolutionary procedure a success. Gray told NPR in an interview that the crippling pain she experienced before CRISPR hasn't returned since the procedure the year before, and she hasn't had any sickle cell–related hospitalizations, emergency room visits, or blood transfusions. Her doctors confirmed that her cells are producing the new version of hemoglobin at a level higher than what they expected would be needed to minimize the sickle cell symptoms.

The results for Victoria Gray and five patients with beta thalassemia who underwent similar CRISPR procedures are giving researchers and patients hope that these blood diseases can be cured entirely in the future by precise editing of the genome. But blood disorders have been just the first step.

Leber congenital amaurosis (LCA) is an eye disease that is a leading cause of blindness in infants. It can be caused by any one of numerous mutations in more than ten genes and primarily affects the retina of the eye. Because researchers had identified the specific mutations that are responsible for LCA, the idea of being able to reverse the blindness, allowing patients to regain some level of sight, with CRISPR seemed reasonable.

Doctors at Oregon Health & Science University's Casey Eye Institute are trying just that. Instead of removing the patient's own cells and then using CRISPR to precisely snip out the genetic variant—the procedure that the patients with sickle cell disease and beta thalassemia underwent—this patient had the CRISPR solution injected directly into one of his eyes. If this method works as well as it did for Victoria Gray, CRISPR could be the vision-saving tool patients with blindness need. Early news from the doctors who performed the procedure say sight improved in the eye that underwent the CRISPR technique, but that had a surprising positive impact on the other eye as well—in 78 percent of the patients!

It's easy to understand why inherited genetic diseases are of so much interest to companies working on CRISPR technologies. After all, if the scientists have identified the mutations that cause the disorders, it isn't conceptually hard to see the benefit of cutting out the mutation and replacing it with the correct nucleotide of DNA. But let's take this idea one step further: why not use it to attack cancer?

First, it's important to remember that some cancer syndromes are inherited. Breast and ovarian cancer syndrome, which can lead to breast, ovarian, and some other cancers, is caused by mutations in the *BRCA1* and *BRCA2* genes. Using CRISPR to "fix" these mutations could be very similar to using the gene-editing tool for sickle cell diseases or even LCA. What's more, this could be done at an early-enough age that the patient hasn't developed the cancer. Instead of worrying about surveillance and extra screening procedures and hoping that the doctors will catch a cancer at an early stage or undergoing life-altering surgeries like removal of ovaries or radical mastectomies in hopes of preventing the cancer, patients could have their mutations CRISPR'ed away.

What about cancers that aren't inherited, but might arise because of exposure to carcinogens, chemicals that cause cancer? That's a more difficult scientific puzzle. Unlike inherited cancers, these might arise from any number of mutations across dozens of genes, from tumor suppressors that fail to stop early cancers in their tracks to growth factor genes that no longer respond to stimuli to shut off, leaving tumors to grow out of control. Targeting the CRISPR machinery before the cancer is detectable is a little like looking for a needle in a three-billion-grain haystack. Instead, scientists hope to use CRISPR alongside another cancer-fighting treatment: immunotherapy.

In a very small Phase I clinical trial at the University of Pennsylvania, doctors combined CRISPR with immunotherapy to treat three very ill cancer patients who failed to respond to other treatments. This early study is more of a proof of principle—can doctors deliver the CRISPR-immunotherapy combination and will the patients tolerate it?—than a test of how well it worked. And in truth, one of the patients died and two patients received additional cancer treatment even after the CRISPR-immunotherapy cocktail. But for a first attempt, this study is nothing short of groundbreaking and offers patients with cancer a glimpse into a future where doctors can precisely treat their cancer by targeting the specific mutations in their tumors.

Are You Ready for the Future?

In this chapter, we've seen how understanding the code behind the DNA is making a difference in health and well-being today, and what it might look like in the future. From newborn sequencing to pharmacogenomics to cancer care, being able to pinpoint specific mutations and then fix them has the potential to completely erase diseases and give patients a chance to treat cancers that arise. And we can use liquid biopsy to monitor patients noninvasively and regularly—so doctors will know when a treatment is working and when they need to switch to the next drug. All of these technologies rely on the secrets hidden in our DNA—and we now have the keys to the language of life.

Have you gotten your DNA sequenced? As you've seen, the first step to using our genome to improve our health comes from knowing what it already says. Though having your entire genome sequenced is still cost-prohibitive for many (to say nothing of how to interpret all that data!), exome sequencing, which focuses on just the parts of the genome that code for proteins, might be more accessible. Genotyping, which is a technology that looks at hundreds of thousands or even a few million individual points across the genome, is even less expensive. Direct-to-consumer companies, like 23andMe and AncestryDNA (these are only two!), all offer one of these technologies and importantly, help you decode what your DNA says. Newer companies like Nebula Genomics offer DNA sequencing without interpretation—pointing users to a number of companies that perform DNA analysis or even do-it-yourself directions on how to take a peek into your genome. And Color and Helix, two companies that are consumer-facing but involve physicians in the ordering process, are hoping to bring DNA sequencing to the masses. Costs continue to fall dramatically for the technology, and there are a number of companies working on software to make it even easier for the average person to understand what's in his or her DNA.

Getting ready to take a statin for high cholesterol or a new antidepressant? You might want to check with your doctor to see if there's a genetic test that could help prescribe the right dose (or even a different medication) for you.

Pharmacogenomic testing is more widespread than ever, and there are a number of drugs with FDA black box warnings recommending or requiring genetic testing be performed before the patient takes the medication. The Clinical Pharmacogenetics Implementation Consortium (https://cpicpgx.org) is a group of researchers helping to provide doctors with peer-reviewed, curated evidence supporting the use of genetic testing to inform prescribing decisions for certain medications. Though its website is geared toward someone with a medical or scientific background, it's fairly easy to navigate and can show you which medications there's already guidance for.

CHAPTER SIX:

PLOTTING YOUR HEALTH FROM THREE BILLION DATA POINTS

"Data, I think, is one of the most powerful mechanisms for telling stories. I take a huge pile of data and I try to get it to tell stories."—*Steven Levitt, author of* Freakonomics

Raise your hand if you, or someone you know, has cancer.

Is your hand up? With an estimated seventeen million new cancer cases worldwide in 2018, chances are it is. While scientists have made tremendous progress in early diagnosis or treating many forms of cancer, others, like pancreatic or ovarian cancers, remain stubbornly out of reach. But cancer's long-held advantage over humans is finally meeting its match.

All data tells a story. It starts with stories that create patterns in the data. These patterns make predictions possible. And predictions, in the world of healthcare, can make the difference between life and death.

Researchers use big data mined from medical research, electronic health records, and other clinical inputs to establish patterns about our health, such as shared characteristics between patients with the same condition or disease. It's how we originally discovered the link between breast cancer and *BRCA1* mutations in patients with Ashkenazi Jewish ancestry, for example, or smoking and lung cancer.

Now we can take those associations one step further: by applying these patterns to *your* unique data, we can make predictions about whether you might get cancer, think cilantro tastes like soap, or if your now-bald newborn will grow up to have a head full of thick, curly black hair, based on shared characteristics between you and millions of people in the past. This is known as predictive analytics. And it's all made possible by the vast amounts of health and genomic data available—everything from lab test results to DNA sequences to the heart rate captured by your smartwatch or fitness tracker.

Radiology's Big Moment

Nowhere is this process playing out more effectively than in the field of radiology, specifically in imaging for breast cancer. Mammography is one of the most important tools available for breast cancer screening. But some people have breasts that are dense or have other characteristics that make it more difficult for radiologists to separate out a worrisome spot from one that is just a normal variation. And it's impossible to find a cancer mass when it's only a few cells large: the limit of detection using available mammogram technology is about the size of a pencil eraser. Often, patients like this might undergo additional tests, like ultrasound, or repeated biopsies to verify a suspicious area, at some cost and potentially considerable worry to the patient.

MIT computer science researcher Dr. Regina Barzilay is finding out firsthand just how powerful AI can be for this purpose. In 2014, Barzilay was diagnosed with breast cancer, and she had the same thoughts as anyone: Will I survive this? Who will look after my family? But the scientist took her experience one step further and focused her research on methods that could help others get an earlier diagnosis, when cancer is often more easily treated and patient outcomes are better.

Dr. Barzilay wants to use AI to take some of the uncertainty out of mammography. Her lab at MIT took data from 88,994 serial mammograms in more than thirty-nine thousand women (consecutive screening mammograms performed year after year in the same patient) to create machine learning algorithms to predict which patients would develop cancer in the next five years.

It would be like having a crystal ball into your medical future. If the program predicts your chances of having breast cancer in the next five years are highly unlikely—maybe 90 percent less likely than the average person your age—maybe you'll just get a screening mammogram every couple of years, instead of every year. But if the program says you're very likely to develop breast cancer and has pointed out exactly where that cancer will develop? Perhaps you'll get the kind of screening that only high-risk patients get today, with MRI or ultrasound, or have screenings every three or six months instead of a year. Or maybe you could undergo a quick procedure, like a biopsy, to remove the cluster of cells that are precancerous, because radiologists know exactly where to look.

The researchers also wanted to see if they could use AI to improve the classification of patients having dense breasts, a known risk factor for breast cancer, and one that makes mammograms less accurate. Determining if someone has dense breasts is somewhat subjective and can vary from radiologist to radiologist, which means that mammography images from the same person could be interpreted differently, based on whether or not the radiologist indicated the individual had dense breasts. A benefit to using AI would be more accurate classification of dense breasts---which could lead to more precise interpretation of women's mammograms. After their deep learning technique was used, the percent of patients reported as having dense breasts decreased from 47 percent to 41 percent. This is important: the better radiologists are at classifying patients with dense breasts, the more accurately they can predict—even without a deep learning algorithm—what a patient's risk for breast cancer is. The overall goal, to help radiologists identify cancers earlier and at lower stages by improving how we determine who has dense breasts and how to interpret areas of concern from mammograms, seems within reach.

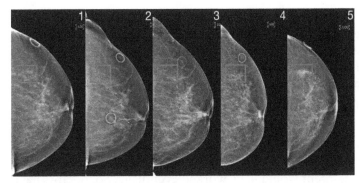

Figure 6.1. Using AI with mammography to detect breast cancer.
[https://www.wired.com/story/doctors-using-ai-screen-breast-cancer/]

The Heart of the Matter

It's not just breast cancer that is getting an assist from AI. Machine learning is being used in other areas of medical testing and for other conditions, including heart disease.

Heart failure affects roughly 6.2 million Americans, with approximately one million new cases in patients fifty-five and older. Symptoms of heart failure include shortness of breath, chronic cough, extreme tiredness or weakness, and sometimes swelling of your ankles or feet. Like cancer, heart failure severity is staged: patients with Stage A (the lowest stage) have pre-heart failure and are at high risk of developing the disease, while those who have Stage D (the highest) have advanced heart failure. Once a patient has a heart failure, the disease severity (how the heart performs or other symptoms) is staged by NYHA class (Classes I–IV). In Class I, patients have few, if any, symptoms when performing normal activities. Patients in Class IV have symptoms like shortness of breath or painful angina, even while they are resting. Treatment options depend on the stage of disease and the severity.

For patients with specific kinds of severe heart failure, one treatment option is a procedure called cardiac resynchronization therapy, where doctors implant a small pacemaker in the heart to help it pump blood more effectively. This works because it causes the heart's out-of-sync ventricles to coordinate their movements, helping the heart to beat more normally again. The benefit to the patient is fewer hospitalizations and lower risk of heart-failure death.

But about a third of patients who receive this treatment don't see an improvement over time in how well their heart is working, and some die too soon to tell if the treatment would have worked eventually. So, doctors have an interest in making sure the right patients are selected for the procedure—identifying who will benefit and survive long enough to see improvement—and patients have an interest in avoiding the risks and costs involved with a surgical procedure that won't end up improving their disease anyway.

Enter machine learning.

Researchers used data from patients with heart failure in Massachusetts to build machine learning algorithms that would predict which patients would see no benefit from cardiac resynchronization therapy. They looked at data from a group of patients who had the treatment and had follow-up information so that they could determine who had, in the end, benefited from the procedure and who had not. In their model, they included data such as medications the patients took, their lab values, if they were male or female, how old patients were at the time of the implant, and information about their heart function from cardiology reports.

From looking at the long-term outcomes from the patients, the researchers knew that ~41 percent either died or had no improvement in their heart's function up to eighteen months after the implant. That means that the doctors' accuracy in selecting the best candidates for the procedure was about 59 percent.

What the researchers wanted to do was find a way to flag the nonresponders—something that would ideally happen before they underwent the procedure—so that both the doctors and the patients could learn the odds of the treatment working and make decisions about whether or not to proceed. The model correctly pointed out patients with reduced benefit from treatment 79 percent of the time—a pretty significant improvement over current methods.

That isn't the only example of machine learning being used to help patients with heart disease. Compared to current guidelines that are used to predict a patient's risk for cardiovascular disease (CVD), machine learning models were able to improve classification of patients (who is going to develop CVD and who isn't). These results have real-life application to patients like you and me. If your doctor could tell you at age twenty-five, thirty-five, or even forty-five how likely you were to develop CVD, and what you could do now to prevent it, wouldn't you want to know?

Detangling Dementia

If you're lucky enough to live to old age, there's about a one-in-fifteen chance of developing Alzheimer's disease, the most common cause of dementia. It's no wonder that so many of us know someone who suffers from the condition. While much has been learned about the disease, the ability to accurately diagnose Alzheimer's in its earliest stages and to offer a cure remain stubbornly out of reach.

Neuroimaging is poised to take advantage of the AI and machine learning revolution that has impacted radiology for other procedures like mammography. Although taking pictures of the brain with a CT scan or MRI might not be technically difficult anymore, interpreting the massive amounts of information can be. Like cardiovascular disease, how can doctors be sure exactly which characteristics are important in the development of dementia and which aren't? Or to classify patients by the type of dementia they have? There's an astronomical number of permutations and combinations of patient characteristics, lab values, and number of neurons in the brain, etc.—too much information for humans to make sense of alone.

While some of the research using machine or deep learning is focused on understanding the mechanics of dementia (how the disease starts and progresses), there is a lot of excitement about using the technologies for early and accurate diagnosis and disease progression. One of the most pressing questions is how we can predict who will get dementia and who won't. While studies over the last few decades have uncovered some insights, like rare susceptibility genes, that question is largely unanswered.

Researchers studied data collected from South Korean senior citizens on the country's National Health Information System database by using a neural network to find risk factors for dementia that are different between men and women, and they identified new ones—characteristics that hadn't been previously associated with the risk of developing dementia. For example, the highest risk for dementia among the men in their cohort was a diagnosis code for psychological problems due to brain damage and physical disease; vitamin D deficiency was third-highest. In women, stroke was the strongest risk factor—something that didn't even crack the top ten for men, while vitamin D deficiency wasn't in the top ten for women.

Why is this important? Imagine your doctor being able to tailor a conversation about dementia based on risk factors that are relevant to you. If you're a man, your risk factors could look very different than those for a woman. But gender might not be the only difference to consider. There could be differences based on any number of things, from the kind of job you have to where you live. Whether vitamin D deficiency is confirmed to be a risk factor for Alzheimer's disease in the future is unclear, but the point is that doctors can't possibly know all of the factors that are important—making the machine learning techniques essential to discovery.

Being able to group patients by the severity of their disease is important, for prognosis (What can they expect next?) and treatment (What medications or clinical trials are they eligible for?). Scientists used machine learning to group patients by their level of cognitive decline based on a combination of characteristics like their gray and white matter volumes—types of brain tissue. They identified a number of brain measurements from MRI scans that were particular to severity, from normal cognitive function to patients with mild cognitive impairment to patients with Alzheimer's disease.

Even though imaging tests like positron emission tomography (PET) scans can identify certain bundles of proteins that are the hallmarks of Alzheimer's disease, they are expensive and not every patient will have access to a hospital or medical center that does the test. This is why definitive diagnosis of Alzheimer's disease currently can only be made after death through examination of the brain. A less invasive, less expensive blood test capable of accurately diagnosing the different types of dementia would be a huge win for patients everywhere.

Another group of scientists, this time in Taiwan, looked for blood-based biomarkers, specific molecules that could be tested with a blood sample, to classify patients with different types of dementia and other neurodegenerative disorders, including Parkinson's disease. They found levels of multiple biomarkers, including ones known to be associated with Alzheimer's disease, tracked with the patient groups. For example, tau protein levels were highest in patients with frontotemporal dementia (a dementia that affects the part of your brain behind your forehead), but alpha-synuclein levels were the highest in Parkinson's disease patients with dementia.

Identifying new risk factors, faster and more accurate diagnoses, and better prognoses by classifying

patients with similar disease trajectories: this is what
machine learning methods are doing to untangle dementia.

The Eyes Have It

Diabetic retinopathy is a type of eye disease that is
a complication of diabetes and is a leading cause of
blindness in adults and affects nearly ten million
Americans. Patients who suffer from diabetic retinopathy
see floaters or spots in their field of vision (Figure 6.2). As
with many diseases, how quickly a person progresses from
minor impairment to complete blindness varies
substantially. This variation is of interest to doctors who
would like to be able to accurately predict which patients
will progress rapidly and which ones will have a lengthier
course. Enter AI.

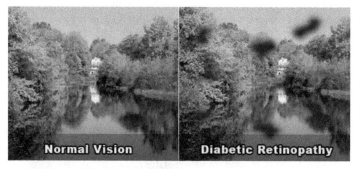

Figure 6.2. What vision looks like to a person with diabetic
retinopathy.
[https://ciplamed.com/content/diabetic-retinopathy-4]

Using deep learning models on photographs of
patients' eyes, researchers were able to predict which
patients would get worse over time. Interestingly, the deep
learning algorithms included both the central and
peripheral retinal areas. This has clinical implications for
patients, because current practice typically involves
photographing only the central retinal area.
Other deep learning models have been developed using the
vast amounts of existing imaging data. In fact, because

patients with this and other eye diseases see their healthcare providers fairly often, each patient might generate multiple eye photographs every year. And these images, combined into large data sets, are what make AI prediction models possible.

Although still emerging, the evidence is compelling that AI models to predict progression of diabetic retinopathy work well. Across eleven such studies, sensitivity of the models ranged from 80 to 100 percent, and accuracy reported by two studies were around 80 percent. And diabetic retinopathy is just one eye-related disorder benefiting from the power of AI. Doctors working on age-related macular degeneration and glaucoma, also leading contributors to blindness worldwide, are using AI methods to better predict progression risk for their patients too.

The Future You: How Much Do You Want to Know?

If a computer algorithm could predict when you were going to die, or from what, would you want to know? That's not just some philosophical question for academics to argue over or a dystopian look at some future world—it's already possible. But instead of filling us with dread or pushing us into an existential crisis, it's giving us a unique opportunity to prepare for that time, and maybe—just maybe—moving us toward a longer, happier healthspan.

In the picturesque, rural town of Danville, Pennsylvania, lies Geisinger Medical Center, one of the nation's top hospitals and part of the larger Geisinger organization, with its thirteen hospitals, two research centers, and medical school. While Geisinger might look on the outside like any other regional hospital, its research arm and medical school keep it competitive with such heavy hitters as Stanford and Harvard. Research at Geisinger focuses a lot of attention on public health research and finding the best ways to care for the more than three million residents who live in central and eastern

Pennsylvania who use its services—including identifying high-risk patients.

Dr. Brandon Fornwalt, a physician-scientist at Geisinger, leads the Cardiac Imaging Technology Laboratory. He and his colleagues at the lab integrate new methods, including machine learning, with more traditional technologies, like electrocardiograms (ECGs). ECGs have been used by doctors for decades to diagnose patients with heart disease or as part of a larger clinical workup to identify patients for interventions, like the cardiac resynchronization therapy I described earlier, but the process isn't perfect.

Some machine learning or AI algorithms can rightfully be said to be like a "black box"—where scientists feed data in and the computer spits out an answer—but no one really knows how the computer got to the solution. This isn't one of those times.

The Geisinger group pulled more than two hundred variables—pieces of data—from the electronic health record: things like height, weight, sex, whether or not someone smoked, and their blood pressure, lab values (like cholesterol levels), and many ECG measurements. The group also included items it called "care gap variables." The eight care gaps represented potential medical interventions that might make a difference in someone's overall health, such as having a flu vaccine, keeping blood pressure in check, or maintaining A1C (blood sugar level) below 8 percent if the individual is diabetic.

The researchers tested several machine learning algorithms for their accuracy in predicting death within a year in patients with heart failure. Though it may seem morbid, doctors already have a variety of models to help them predict someone's survival (or the converse, mortality)—usually on a short time scale, like one or two years. The Seattle Heart Failure Model (SHFM) is one and predicts survival/mortality and life expectancy over one, two, and five years in patients with heart failure. The

Charlson Comorbidity Index is another, which predicts ten-year survival in patients with multiple health issues.

Next, they evaluated two different clinical models: one where the care gap variables were exactly as it was reported in the medical record, and one where the care gap was closed. For example, choosing not to receive a flu shot or keeping blood pressure under control in the first model, and then a new model where flu vaccine was received and blood pressure was good. When they compared the results of the two models, they predicted that closing those care gaps reduced overall one-year mortality—the impact of 231 additional patients surviving another year.

Doctors already know that maintaining a healthy weight or blood glucose level is important for overall well-being and survival. But most humans can only keep so much information at a time in our heads—think about the largest string of numbers you can rattle off without thought. Maybe a phone number (including area code, ten digits)? The doctors in this study included more than two hundred different variables—a feat beyond human capability—or the average office visit.

The ability of computers to mesh all of the data together and figure out what is crucial and what isn't for an individual patient's survival is what will make AI and machine learning an essential part of healthcare. Imagine a doctor being able to tell you that your chances of living another year would double, triple, or more, if you'd just get the flu vaccine, or make sure you are taking your blood pressure medicine correctly, while your neighbor might need to switch to a different arthritis medication and keep his or her A1C level below 7 percent.

Sometimes, AI and machine learning models are like the proverbial black box: doctors know what goes into them but can't figure out how the computer spits out the answer. Research out of Dr. Fornwalt's lab using AI-enabled computers forecast with uncanny accuracy who might die of a heart condition within a year's time in more than two hundred fifty thousand patients, including those whose ECGs were deemed healthy by their doctors, is a case in point. They just aren't entirely sure what the computer is picking up as a risk factor.

In this study, Dr. Fornwalt and his colleagues took nearly 1.8 million ECGs from almost four hundred thousand patients collected over thirty-four years in the Geisinger system and applied a deep neural network (see Chapter One) to predict one-year mortality. Not only was the prediction from their model better than existing ones; it also uncovered significant differences in clinical measurements between patients who survived and those who were deceased. This has substantial value for clinical care.

Finally, the researchers wanted to see if cardiologists, using traditional methods, could find diagnostic features in the same ECGs that the computer model used. To do this, they took 802 ECGs, 401 each of patients who survived and who died, that the computer model correctly identified. Each pair of ECGs was assessed by three cardiologists to see if they could correctly identify which patient survived by looking at the ECG. The cardiologists performed little better than random chance alone. Even after the researchers showed the cardiologists ECGs where the outcome was labeled, their accuracy on the original 802 ECGs was about the same. So somehow, the computer is pulling out features that trained cardiologists can't find—with far better accuracy.

Many of the computer models using AI and machine learning are focused on outcomes in patients with heart disease. This isn't really unexpected: these patients are regularly seen by their doctors, are often hospitalized for procedures or because of disease complications, and have tests, like ECGs, that provide enormous amounts of data that can be used to develop these models. Other conditions or diseases, like cancer, where imaging data is used to monitor disease and treatment progress, are also ripe for an overhaul using AI and machine learning.

And the "black box" models of AI may be a thing of the past—at some point. The Explainable Machine Learning Challenge was a 2018 competition where teams created a complicated AI model and had to explain how it worked. Sounds relatively simple, and for some machine learning models, like the one used by Dr. Fornwalt's team to identify the care gaps that predicted patients' survival, researchers know what variables turned out to be important and which weren't. For others, like the ECG study above, we sometimes have no clue what the machine is picking up that human eyes can't.

The Challenge had an unusual twist: one of the teams created a model that they could fully explain—they knew exactly how it was working—which drove the organizers to ask, "Why are we using black box models in AI when we don't need to?" It's a great question.

Are You Ready for the Future?

In this chapter, I've shown how innovative doctors and scientists are embracing a new paradigm of healthcare, where man and machines work together more closely than ever before. We've seen how imaging tests, like mammograms, do better at finding very-early-stage cancers when human interpretation is paired with AI algorithms that point out areas of concern. Although some of this research is still in early stages, there are already some places where AI- and machine learning–enabled healthcare is changing patients' lives for the better.

So what can you do today?

- Worried about cancer? In addition to helping doctors with imaging, machine learning and AI can combine hundreds, thousands, or even more data points to find out which patients are at risk for cancer or another disease, and which patients will stay healthy. These prediction models are still mostly in early stages, except for when there's a reasonably strong genetic component (like

BRCA1 or *BRCA2* and breast cancer). All of these models rely on massive amounts of data to improve their accuracy—everything from correct family history to recent blood tests.

There are several things you can do if you're worried about cancer—many of them decidedly low-tech. Putting together an accurate family medical history may be one of the most important things you can do to help your doctors get a better understanding of your inherited risks for some cancers. Sharing work-related information, like whether you are exposed to certain chemicals, is also valuable.

- Do your doctors and your local hospital perform research using de-identified or anonymized data from electronic health records? You might be asked if researchers can use your data to further the kinds of research I've described. Data found in EHRs, from lab tests to procedure information to X-ray and other imaging reports, are what help researchers like Dr. Barzilay and Dr. Fornwalt make their incredible discoveries—so the more data that can be used, the better these algorithms can be.

- Wonder what the benefits are of predictive algorithms or predictive tests for conditions where there is no cure? This is a common question— after all, why would someone want to know if he or she is going to get Alzheimer's disease or ALS when existing treatments fall far short of a cure? Many folks would rather not know, to avoid the stress and anxiety that knowledge would bring. But for those who would rather have a chance to prepare for the inevitable, predictive algorithms could be just what they need to put their affairs in order, change their jobs, or start knocking off their bucket lists. And even though we may not have a cure for some conditions today, there's no telling how much more we'll know in five or ten years. With medical advances and innovations occurring at such a rapid-fire pace, it's not unthinkable that conquering these conditions could happen in our lifetimes.

CHAPTER SEVEN:

DRUG DISCOVERY'S AI MOMENT

"There is no medicine like hope, no incentive so great, and no tonic so powerful as expectation of something tomorrow." —*Orison Swett Marden, nineteenth-century inspirational author*

Who among us wouldn't prefer to have an outpatient surgery that gets you back to your normal life in days versus a complicated surgical procedure that keeps you in the hospital with a long recovery? Or the ability to take a pill for six weeks to cure your illness that has virtually no side effects compared to one you have to take for six months that leaves you feeling miserable and unable to enjoy family or your favorite activities? How about lower medication costs or to finally have a cure for diseases like Alzheimer's?

We've already seen how AI is helping doctors to diagnose diseases (see Chapters Five and Six)—with the goal to identify and treat the patient earlier in the disease, when the medication or procedure is often less invasive, has fewer side effects, and is more easily tolerated. And we've seen a glimpse of how you might receive treatment, from telemedicine to futuristic hospitals with command centers like spaceship holodecks (Chapter Four). In this chapter, I'll show you how scientists are using the power of AI to discover new drugs and find new uses for existing ones.

Data-driven software is helping scientists and researchers discover new cures and significantly shorten the time from drug discovery to prescription-ready. AI-enabled computers that can mine medical studies, existing drug libraries, and millions of compounds that may treat or cure a condition, eliminate years of research and the billions of dollars it often takes to develop a drug—the cost of which is usually passed down to the patient. Researchers can also use AI to better pinpoint the root causes of disease, allowing them to develop drugs that successfully target the condition at its molecular level.

When it comes to clinical testing, AI also saves time and money by allowing pharmaceutical companies to develop statistical models that can determine whether a drug will work even before the treatment goes to trial. When 90 percent of all drugs currently fail before even hitting the market, getting the medication to the right patients is a big (and expensive) deal.

The more treatments and cures for medical conditions that AI finds, the more lives the technology can help extend and save. For this reason, drug development is one of the most exciting areas in AI right now. For proof, just look at the coronavirus outbreak: AI was instrumental in helping scientists discover which drug molecules could kill the virus (see more about this in Chapter Eight). And scientists are using deep learning approaches to find new antibiotics—essential for the growing number of "superbugs" that existing antibiotics can't kill. What's perhaps even more important, many of the large databases used to help researchers discover new applications for existing drugs are already publicly available. That's important, because other scientists can use that information to help them avoid going down rabbit holes and chasing dead ends—saving everyone time and money.

If a therapy appears promising for trial, the process of recruiting patients for a clinical study will also be quicker and more effective with AI. The advent of smartphone medicine and electronic health records has already made it easier for drug manufacturers to identify ideal patients and recruit them. Additionally, trials can be conducted virtually, increasing a study's efficiency and possible participant pool. Many clinical trials also now rely on smartphone apps, wearable sensors, and other AI-enabled devices to collect continuous, accurate, real-world feedback, which is more reliable than episodic information or subjective data reported by patients. Together, this is increasing the efficacy of treatments while lowering the cost and time it takes from discovery to approved use.

The Data Deluge

Now that patient records are digital (you can even access your chart from your smartphone, in some cases), doctors are now faced with the enormity of the data. Each interaction with a patient, from an in-person or telehealth visit, to a hospital stay, to getting blood drawn, adds to the overall patient record. This is good; we need and want to be better at capturing these encounters and having a record of them for both accounting and patient care. But it can be difficult to quickly access the information you need in these large EHR systems, which were designed originally for use as accounting systems. Researchers don't need all of the insurance and billing information and are mostly focused on narrow research questions. Physicians investigating the use of blood thinners in their geriatric population don't want to sift through pediatric records (wrong population) or patients not taking the medication (wrong intervention).

It's not just medications and ICD codes that are behind this overwhelming amount of data. In Chapter Five, I described the AI systems that were trained to identify very early breast cancers using mammograms. Those mammograms and other medical imaging contribute to the deluge of data. Every X-ray, CT scan, and MRI are not just one data point, but hundreds, thousands, or millions.

It's not only doctors who are faced with the growing quagmire of information. Researchers working to discover new drugs are constantly trying to manage data that emerges from new studies and clinical trials, the growing number of compounds in chemical screening databases, models of chemical structures, and how compounds interact with any number of other substances. The sheer amount of information is overwhelming.

Sidebar:
How Big Is Your Brain?

Let's take the average brain MRI, like one you might have for recurrent migraine headaches. The MRI takes a 3D view of the brain; just like a two-dimensional object can be located precisely on a coordinate system, so can every neuron or flash of electrical impulse of the brain in a 3D coordinate system. If you divide the brain into tiny cubes, each cube is called a voxel (Figure 7.1).

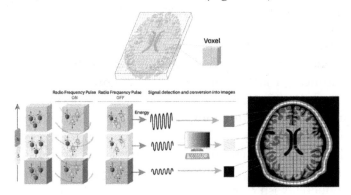

Figure 7.1. MRI scans and voxels.
[https://knowingneurons.com/2017/09/27/mri-voxels/]

The size of the voxel depends on the type of MRI being used: a standard MRI voxel is 1 mm^3 (meaning 1mm on each side of the cube), while a functional MRI voxel is generally larger and varies by the study. If the brain takes up one hundred eight thousand voxels, and the researcher wants to measure the effect of a drug over time on specific neurons, each time point (minutes, seconds, or tiny fractions of a second) gets multiplied by the number of voxels. So, if you're comparing what happens at each voxel for sixty seconds, you now have more than six million voxels to analyze! Now, think about the amount of data created by a study that enrolled fifty patients, or where the MRI took a picture of the brain each second for an hour. It's not just a data deluge—it's a data tsunami!
—End Sidebar—

Computer, Heal Thyself

You might think that having all this data is a good thing for doctors and researchers—and to a point, it is. We definitely do not want to go back to the days of paper charts with limited functionality or notebooks full of yellowing journal articles with hand-scribbled notes in the margins. But the larger the data sets are, and the more information you try to analyze, the more computational resources are required. If you've ever worked with a really large spreadsheet with dozens of columns and tens of thousands of rows and tried to calculate a figure, you've probably encountered the "curse of dimensionality." As you add data, it takes longer and longer for the computer to crunch through it, and there can be more uncertainty in the results. You can see in Figure 7.2 that performance quickly drops off the more data you have. Because each column and row adds another dimension, when we're talking about the enormous amounts of data in EHRs or other medical and scientific databases, that drop-off in productivity isn't trivial.

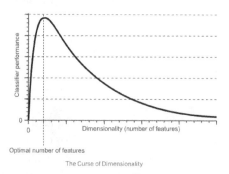

Figure 7.2. The Curse of Dimensionality.
(https://www.visiondummy.com/wp-content/uploads/2014/04/dimensionality_vs_performance.png)

Managing dimensionality can be done manually— let's say for our project looking at blood thinners in the elderly, we can drop any data that is thought to be irrelevant and focus only on those variables that are important: other medications the person is taking, any procedures they may have had in the last five years. But this can be time-consuming and requires that the person doing the task has correctly figured out which variables are important and which ones are safe to ignore. It's probably not difficult to imagine a scenario where a variable is mistakenly removed.

But why not just task the computer with figuring out on its own which data points can be safely removed? That's exactly what "dimensionality reduction" aims to do. When we have the computer figure out which variables are important and which aren't for a specific outcome, we can sometimes find surprising connections (or a lack thereof) between things we humans didn't even suspect!

What's more, by reducing the number of dimensions, we can speed up the computational processes, getting us to an answer sooner. When it comes to analyzing the vast amounts of imaging, laboratory, and clinical data found in EHRs, dimensionality reduction is essential to helping researchers get a handle on the data deluge facing them. And these machine learning techniques are used by nearly every industry—not just healthcare or science. Back in Chapter One, I explained how companies are using this to get a handle on the kind of consumer you are and selectively offer you products or services you are likely the most interested in.

Big Pharma's Time and Money Problems

How much money do you think it takes a pharmaceutical company to bring the average drug from initial discovery all the way through FDA approval so it can be marketed and prescribed? $10 million? $100 million? A billion dollars? How long do you think that process takes? Five years? Ten? How many drugs that a pharmaceutical company tests actually make it all the way to the finish line?

Would you guess three-quarters? Half? Less than 25 percent?

Would it surprise you to learn that a 2016 study from the Tufts Center for the Study of Drug Development found that when all the pre- and post-FDA approval costs for research and development were added up, it costs roughly $2.8 billion to bring a drug to market? That from test tube to your pharmacy the process can take more than a decade? And that the rate of success can be as little as 5 percent for some drug classes? The high prices we pay for medications aren't a big surprise when put into that context.

What drug companies need are ways to minimize the enormous risks they take when deciding to develop a new drug. A way of pushing the needle toward more successes and fewer failures. A method that could shave months or even years off the timeline. Something that could reduce their investments in drugs that might not even make it to market.

Alzheimer's disease is a perfect example. Alzheimer's is a devastating neurodegenerative disease that causes dementia. In Chapter Six, I described how advances in AI are helping doctors better identify what type of dementia someone has, earlier than ever before, with AI-assisted interpretation of brain scans. But even as diagnosis improves, a cure for Alzheimer's remains stubbornly out of reach.

One of the most important findings scientists have discovered are tangles of proteins, beta-amyloid and tau, that build up in the brain and are characteristic of Alzheimer's. The disease appears to always follow the same path: first the beta-amyloid protein aggregates in the brain. Next, tau protein appears, the proteins tangle up, and the patient's neurons begin to die, causing the symptoms of dementia. As scientific thinking goes, if you can stop the beta-amyloid from accumulating in the brain in the first place, you should be able to stop the tau protein from appearing and halt the progression of dementia. It's common sense.

Naturally, then, most clinical trials in the past two decades have targeted the beta-amyloid protein—only to fail a staggering 99 percent of the time! What can be done about the billions of dollars down the drain and the countless families whose hopes for a cure are dashed time and again?

Big Data (and AI) to the Rescue

Drug companies certainly don't want to throw away research dollars on drugs that won't be prescribed, nor do scientists want to waste their time on experiments that lead nowhere. This is the kind of problem that AI and machine learning can excel with.

For example, let's take (nearly) everyone's favorite molecule: caffeine. We know that its molecular formula $C_8H_{10}N_4O_2$ means that each molecule of caffeine has eight carbon atoms, ten of hydrogen, four of nitrogen, and two of oxygen. We know the shape of the caffeine molecule and, using that, can figure out how it physically interacts with other compounds. But there are an incomprehensible number of molecules, just like caffeine, waiting to be identified or even created in a lab, each with an unimaginable number of interactions with other chemicals and effects on plants, animals, and humans. The human brain can't keep track of every compound or molecule that's been discovered or created, and what effect it has. But computers can, and the results can be surprising.

Researchers can feed every piece of information about every chemical ever discovered into databases that AI and machine learning systems can go through. Sifting through these massive databases, the systems "learn" to categorize the molecules—sometimes grouping them in ways that are completely surprising to researchers who couldn't see the underlying patterns tying them together. This is one of the ways scientists have figured out that drugs developed for one disease might work on a completely unrelated condition. (In Chapter Eight, I'll describe how drugs developed for leprosy found new interest for treating COVID-19.)

It's not just chemicals that machine learning and AI can work their magic on. Remember the Alzheimer's problem, where study after study focused on the beta-amyloid and tau protein tangles? In 2018, the media was buzzing about findings from a study led by Dr. Joel Dudley, then at the Icahn School of Medicine at Mount Sinai in New York City. In a *New York Times* interview, Dr. Dudley said, "'I went looking for drugs, and all I found were these stupid viruses."

Instead of focusing their attention on the much-studied proteins, Dr. Dudley and his colleagues decided to let the computer figure out what was important using machine learning techniques. Dr. Dudley's lab compared the genomes and viral makeup of brain samples from patients with late-stage Alzheimer's to those who did not have the disease. The result? The scientists found more evidence of common viruses, specifically herpesviruses, in patients with Alzheimer's disease than in patients without the disorder—an idea that had been tossed around by a few scientists over the years, but without gaining any real traction. Though Dr. Dudley was quick to point out that the findings didn't show that having a virus caused Alzheimer's, the results generated a lot of interest in the idea that there could be another target for clinical trials and helped move the virus-Alzheimer's connection from a fringe theory more to the mainstream. There are even ongoing clinical trials looking at treating patients who have Alzheimer's disease with antiviral medications.

Why is this important to the average person? Well, while scientists use the peer-review process to weed out theories that lead nowhere, it's still possible to get hung up on an idea based on the data at hand—which might be incomplete. So, even though researchers have a pretty good idea how the protein tangles lead to dementia and

Alzheimer's symptoms, and it made sense to focus attention on drugs that could stop beta-amyloid or tau proteins in the first place, after countless studies, it is pretty clear that scientists are barking up the wrong tree, and there are still some missing parts to the puzzle that they haven't been able to crack (yet). Letting a machine sort through the thousands of studies that have been published on the disease, everything from basic research using mice and cell lines to the large-scale Phase III clinical trials, we stand a better chance of discovering new connections between diseases and their causes and treatments without scientists having to narrow the scope first. That saves researchers crucial time and the taxpayers and corporations that fund this research billions of dollars.

A New Kind of Clinical Trial

I've explained how using AI or machine learning can help to target the most promising new drugs to treat diseases, but what happens next? As a consequence of the COVID-19 pandemic, the words "clinical trial" recently entered many people's conversations. Before COVID-19, if you asked the average person what a clinical trial was, they would probably respond that it had something to do with cancer treatments. That's definitely a big part of what clinical trials are for—but they are used for any new drug, procedure, or medical device before it's approved by the FDA for widespread use.

Preclinical, or Phase 0, studies are the experiments that happen before something is tested in humans. These are the experiments done at a lab bench using cells in test tubes or petri dishes, in model organisms like worms, zebrafish, or mice, and possibly a very small (under fifteen) group of people. This is where the scientific theory gets tested, like a proof-of-concept: Does new Drug A have the desired effect when tested in a mouse model of disease? Does it appear that the drug could be safe at a very small dose to give to humans? It's impossible to say just how many of these preclinical experiments are done—but it's a lot—and this is one of the first places that AI and machine learning can help to narrow down the choices and focus on the most promising candidates.

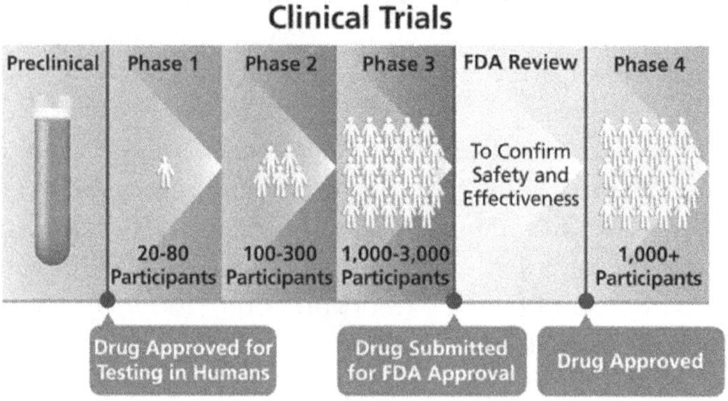

Clinical Trials

Figure 7.3. The pathway from lab experiment to FDA-approved drug. (https://onlinesciencenotes.com/different-phases-of-clinical-trials-drugs-testing-and-development-of-vaccines-in-clinical-research/)

Once there have been sufficient preclinical studies and there is enough interest to move on, the drug will be tested in a small number of actual patients, typically somewhere between twenty and eighty, in Phase I trials (Figure 7.3). The goal here isn't to see how well it performs; it's to make sure that the drug can be safely tested in more people and figure out the best way of getting into the body and what the dose should be. These trials generally last only a few months. Participants in Phase I trials are very closely monitored, and any adverse event that occurs will be very closely scrutinized. The probability of a drug moving from Phase I to Phase II was estimated to be roughly 66 percent in a 2018 study. While that doesn't sound so bad, across all kinds of drugs for any disease or condition, the likelihood of success—that is, getting from Phase I all the way through to FDA approval—was less than 7 percent!

If the drug is considered to be tolerated and succeeded in Phase I trials, it will move on to Phase II. These trials include up to several hundred people with the disorder, and the focus is on how effective the drug is and what side effects occur. Phase II trials last longer than Phase I—up to a few years—so that researchers can be fairly confident that any side effects from the drug have had time to appear in their study population and to see if the drug's effectiveness remains high or only lasts a short time. While the probability of a drug successfully moving to Phase III is less than 50 percent now, the overall probability of a Phase II drug getting FDA approval increases.

Phase III clinical trials are the ones most people are familiar with. These are large studies that can enroll thousands of volunteers and that often take place at multiple locations simultaneously. Phase III trials are also the longest—taking several years to complete—as the researchers continue to evaluate how effective the drug is for the condition and monitor any side effects that occur.

Though it may seem unnecessary to have Phase III trials if Phase II ones have been completed successfully, it's actually very important. Not every person who takes a medication will have the same side effects (if any) as another person taking it. The larger enrollment in Phase III trials gives researchers a better chance at seeing side effects that might be somewhat rare and only affect one in a thousand or one in five thousand patients who take the drug. In Phase II studies with a few hundred people, those rare side effects would be unlikely to pop up. If a drug makes it through Phase III studies, its odds of ultimately getting approved by the FDA are pretty good—about 60 percent. But this varies tremendously, based on the type of drug/medication/compound being tested. For example, a new vaccine's probability of getting approved from the beginning (Phase I) is about 33 percent, or one in three, while cardiovascular drugs only have about a one-in-four chance and cancer drugs only a little more than 3 percent!

What makes the approval rate so low? It's complicated and involves many factors. In the Alzheimer's studies, for example, what looks like a promising drug turns out not to have any effect on the outcome of interest once more people start taking the medication. Or it may turn out that only a small fraction of the intended population will derive some benefit from the medication, while the rest get nothing from it—or worse, have some sort of negative effect. With billions of dollars and years of development on the line, what's a pharmaceutical company to do?

AI to the Rescue (Again)!

There's a lot that advanced analytics using machine learning and AI can do. Here's an overview:

Identifying top drug candidates that are more likely to move from Phase I all the way to FDA approval. Researchers can use computers to play out scenarios of drug-drug interactions and the best targets for the drug. And even when the scientists aren't entirely sure of how a specific new drug could work, they can use machine learning techniques to better classify the drug and figure out its most likely effects based on existing information. So, if a pharmaceutical company wants to develop a new blood pressure–lowering drug, they can use what is already known about drugs currently on the market and those that have failed in the past to guide development.

Beyond simply identifying which drug out of multiple options is the best gamble, pharmaceutical companies can also rely on AI and machine learning algorithms to determine the best dose of the new drug. By getting that right at the outset of Phase I or even the late-stage preclinical trial, it might improve the number of drug candidates making it to Phase II (and all the way to approval) by reducing the number of serious side effects that would spell disaster and the end of the drug study.

Pharmaceutical industry company Aria Pharmaceuticals (formerly twoXAR) is using AI to compress the preclinical steps (searching through the scientific literature, basic science, and high-throughput screening) into a single step. Its unique and rapid technology enabled it to identify and start testing two different drug candidates for treatment of chronic kidney disease in four weeks. That's less time than a review of the existing literature without AI would take by itself!

Identifying the right patients. In Chapter 5, I described the idea behind pharmacogenomics—using genomics and genetic information together with what is known about how the drug is absorbed, metabolized, or excreted, to get the drug to the right patient. It's a key aspect of precision medicine—the idea that medical care can be optimized and personalized for individual patients based on their characteristics, genetic information, and environment. And this is where AI and machine learning can shine in clinical trials. Remember how many clinical trials fail at the last stage, demonstrating little or no effect on the condition, or where the adverse side effects outweigh any benefit? Instead, pharmaceutical companies can identify which patients are most likely to benefit ahead of time and specifically seek those patients for clinical trials. They can also use that information to exclude patients who are highly likely to develop serious problems from taking the drug based on their genetic data.

AI can also help patients find the right clinical trials. Even though thousands of clinical trials are waiting to enroll patients, most will end up failing and shutting down because they can't get enough patients signed up. This is tragedy on multiple fronts: the patients lose out on the opportunity to help science and possibly find a new treatment for their conditions, while the drug companies lose out on their investments of time and money trying to get a clinical trial launched. Much like how consumers can shop for the best price for a vacation package, new companies are turning to AI and machine learning platforms, hoping that doctors and patients will do the same thing to enroll in clinical trials. Imagine getting a new diagnosis and your doctor tells you about this great website that will match you with the perfect clinical trial in seconds. As a patient, having a resource that makes clinical trial participation as simple as possible can be the difference between enrolling or not. And for some diseases where clinical trials offer the best hope for a treatment or cure, getting to the right clinical trial is essential.

How about a clinical trial "digital twin"? What if you could run a clinical trial in half the time it normally takes or with half the number of people? Pharmaceutical companies would be thrilled, and patients could reap the benefits of new medications more quickly. Enter Unlearn.AI, a company based in San Francisco that uses machine learning to create a so-called "digital twin" for clinical trials. The digital twin idea isn't new—it's been used in aerospace engineering to help manufacturers play out how a particular part or piece of machinery, even entire engines or planes, will run over their lifetimes.

It can be difficult to recruit enough patients to run a clinical trial, particularly when the patients all want to be randomized to the experimental treatment. After all, how many of us would say they'd be excited to get the placebo? But patients who get the placebo treatment are incredibly important in clinical trials. They are how we know just how well a drug works—or doesn't.

Using electronic health records or data from actual clinical trials of patients in control groups, Unlearn.AI creates a digital twin of patients in the study with machine learning. These "twins" virtually get the placebo treatment, while the real person gets the experimental drug. While this technique can be used to create an entire cohort of virtual patients who get the placebo in a trial, it can also be added to the data from actual patients. Instead of having to recruit one hundred patients who are randomized to the control group, a pharmaceutical company might only need to find fifty, and use digital twins to fill in the rest.

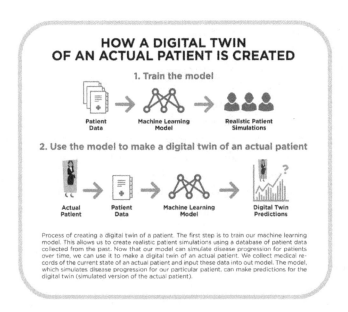

Figure 7.4. Digital Twins for Clinical Trials.
[Adapted from: https://www.unlearn.ai/post/what-is-a-digital-twin]

Can you run a clinical trial in virtual reality or using only connected devices like smartwatches? The answer(s) is yes. I've already explained how virtual reality is being used to help treat chronic pain in place of opioids (see Chapter Three). Ingestibles used to deliver medication or for disease surveillance are being tested for a variety of conditions. As people become increasingly comfortable with connected devices and wearables, expect to see more digital therapeutics used by themselves and alongside medications.

Sidebar:
The Clinical Trial Is in New York, but You're in Wyoming

One of the reasons that otherwise eligible people don't volunteer for clinical trials is that they don't live near a study site. Even though many large clinical trials have multiple sites scattered throughout a region or even across the country, chances are that if you live in a somewhat rural area, you're not likely to be within even an hour's drive of the closest facility. It's a big problem for both patients and drug companies who want to include as many people (and as diverse a population) as they can for their trials.

In addition to any initial exams or procedures that take place at the start of a study, many trials rely on regular visits to the study sites to collect additional information, like an accurate weight or taking your blood pressure exactly two hours after you last ate. But wait. You might be thinking, "Why can't I do this from my house? Or at least go to my regular doctor for the check-ins?"

And you'd be right! Many clinical trials are embracing digital health devices, like smartwatches or connected scales, as a way of capturing real world evidence—how the drug or device works in situations closer to real life versus the very controlled, strict environment of traditional clinical trials. Using these devices or sensors also gives more people an opportunity to participate in trials in the first place. Combined with apps and surveys you can take straight from your smartphone, companies are making it easier than ever to volunteer for a trial, no matter where you live.

This is where companies like Evidation Health are changing the existing clinical trials paradigm. Evidation works with companies to enroll patients from the convenience of their homes using their smartphones. Using surveys and health and fitness data that users on their platform have opted to share, the start-up can provide real-world evidence—that is, data from the average person—for a variety of conditions. This is particularly useful, since populations in clinical trials don't always reflect the average users of devices or medications.

—End Sidebar—

The Future You: Citizen Scientist

In this chapter, we've seen how AI and machine learning are transforming the drug discovery process to get drugs to market more quickly, with better candidates likely to pass the FDA approval hurdles and improve patient participation in clinical trials. Although these technologies are somewhat in their infancy, they're making a big impact already. In the next chapter, you'll learn how they have turned the entire health and wellness industry upside down. And as I'll show you in Chapter Eight, AI and machine learning played a large role in the ability of multiple companies to develop a COVID-19 vaccine in such a short time.

What may be the most important thing to come from AI and machine learning in this space is that the average person can participate in the scientific process without having to spend decades becoming a doctor or scientist. It all comes down to data.

Are You Ready for the Future?

By now, I hope you're convinced that while AI and machine learning might not save the world, they play an enormous role in improving how clinical trials are done, increase the odds that a new drug will make it across the FDA approval finish line, and even reduce the impact of the data deluge healthcare providers and researchers are swimming in. But you don't have to get a degree in data science to personally have an impact and see firsthand how transformative these technologies can be. Here's what you can do today:

Have a smartphone and a smartwatch? That data, captured by your everyday movements, can be incredibly helpful for researchers studying things like exercise and overall activity.

Want to be a citizen scientist? Participating in a clinical trial has never been easier—especially with digital trials and connected devices. By clicking the widget on some websites, like the Type 1 diabetes organization JDRF, and answering a few questions, you'll get information about the nearest clinical trial to you and how to reach out to study coordinators. AI-assisted platforms, like Antidote, are making this matchmaking possible. What's more, you don't have to be sick or have a certain condition or disease to participate—many trials need healthy volunteers.

Want to opt in to a patient study? Connected devices can provide drug companies with real-world evidence, a critical component of Phase IV (post-FDA approval) studies. Consider opting in to these long-term safety and efficacy studies that give manufacturers a look at how the average patient does on a new drug.

CHAPTER EIGHT:

SOLVING THE PANDEMIC PROBLEM

"I cannot imagine a better use of AI." —*Thomas Siebel, founder of C3.ai, on the application of AI to the coronavirus pandemic*

The typical winter and holiday season looks something like this for me: trips across the country to see family, wrapping up work meetings with colleagues for the end of the year, and spending time with my family, enjoying holiday parties with friends, maybe a few ski trips to Maine or—if I am truly lucky—a getaway to a warm, sunny island like Barbados for some needed relaxation and vitamin D. Spring starts off with a bang, and you will find me busy with work-related travel across the country and the globe, and in the summer, a family vacation to visit family in Europe or back in California. Travel and in-person interactions with family, friends, and business colleagues are a given and consistent throughout the year—and with my personality just downright necessary. That all changed in early 2020 for me and countless others.

Instead of spring break trips, we had shelter-in-place recommendations. We watched New York City quickly become the epicenter of the US outbreak, listened to firsthand accounts of medical staff pushed to their limits and beyond as hospital beds and ICU space filled up, leaving the sick with no place to go. We grew accustomed to the White House daily briefing with Dr. Anthony Fauci and other infectious disease experts who taught listeners about viruses, transmission rates, and prevention measures—creating an entire nation of armchair epidemiologists. And as the situation in New York and across the Northeast became less dire in late spring, we watched as other parts of the country faced similar trials throughout the summer, fall, and winter.

The coronavirus pandemic changed nearly every aspect of modern society on a global scale, including how we approach healthcare. Though the consequences have been catastrophic for so many, it also opened the eyes of millions of Americans to the power of AI, with the technology heralded as one of the most effective weapons in the fight against the virus.

From the outbreak's onset, AI played a critical role in helping researchers understand the new virus. The AI-enabled Canadian platform BlueDot, for example, spotted warning signs of the epidemic in Wuhan, China, nine days before the World Health Organization did. Its algorithms also predicted where the virus might travel next, helping officials prepare residents and hospitals.

AI helped researchers sequence the virus's genome in days, not the months it took us to map the SARS genome in 2003. IBM's supercomputer Summit (or OLCF-4) quickly identified seventy-seven drug compounds capable of targeting the virus, helping drug developers explore possible treatments almost immediately. Just days after the outbreak began in the US, dozens of smartphones apps had emerged, including a COVID-19 screening tool, created by Apple and the Centers for Disease Control, that used chatbot technology to help people determine if they had the virus, and whether they needed to go to the emergency room. Other apps followed, including one that detects the virus with 70 percent accuracy from the sound of a cough.

AI-enabled tools also allowed employers to check the temperature of essential employees without any contact and helped people monitor their respiration rate, blood oxygen, and other biomarkers of the illness—from home. AI surveillance devices helped some governments enforce quarantine restrictions for those who tested positive for the virus, while robots sanitized hospitals and drones delivered COVID tests. Data-driven software also helped develop the statistical models that government and health officials relied on to make critical decisions about medical supplies and lockdown policies, and who was likely to develop severe COVID-19 complications during hospitalization. It's hard to imagine just how much worse things could have been without the rapid development of diagnostic tests, vaccines, and treatments.

COVID-19 is just the beginning. In the coming years, scientists predict more outbreaks and pandemics will shake the world, as global populations increase alongside urbanization, climate change, and international travel. This chapter will explore how AI can help thwart and prevent pandemics and perhaps even solve the centuries-old riddle of treating the seasonal flu and common cold.

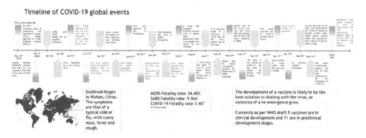

Figure 8.1. A timeline of how AI helped to tame the coronavirus crisis. [https://www.frontiersin.org/articles/10.3389/fpubh.2020.00216/full]

Who Is Patient Zero?

It might be hard to remember back to the first few anxious days and weeks in late December 2019 and early January 2020, when the world was transfixed by the news coming out of China: a new respiratory illness with cases growing exponentially. There was much about the illness that was unknown in the beginning: what caused it, how it was transmitted, and how to stop it. Global public health agencies, like the World Health Organization (WHO), were particularly alarmed, given the severity of the previous SARS and MERS outbreaks (See Figure 8.1), and warned countries to take precautions against the spread of this new illness. But as we know, that advice was not enough to stop the spread of SARS-CoV-2—the virus that causes the disease COVID-19. How can scientists tell who is "Patient Zero"—the first patient to become infected?

This is where the magic of genetics, epidemiology, and computers meets gumshoe detective strategy.

On January 20, 2020, the US saw the first patient diagnosed with the SARS-CoV-2 virus: a middle-aged man living in Snohomish County, north of Seattle, Washington. The patient had recently returned from a trip to visit family in Wuhan, China, and after several days of fever and cough, headed to an urgent care facility on January 19. After tests for the most common respiratory ailments—influenza (flu), rhinovirus (the common cold), respiratory syncytial virus (RSV), and others—came back negative, swabs were taken to be tested for the new SARS-CoV-2 virus. A day later, after the results were positive, the patient was taken to a special isolation room at a regional hospital for observation. Although the first hospital days passed unremarkably, the patient later developed pneumonia—a common complication that had been seen in cases in China. After two weeks of hospitalization, the patient was released. Even as the news reported that the Washington man was the first US patient with the novel coronavirus infection, there were murmurs that the virus had been circulating in the US for some time.

Epidemiologists use contact tracing to help identify Patient Zero. This is a lot like old-fashioned detective work. While epidemiologists in the field might not wear a trench coat and hat or carry around a magnifying glass like in an old detective novel, they painstakingly work backward to identify everyone that a patient may have come into contact with in the days leading up to their illness. When they find who was sick before the current patient, they do the same contact tracing for them, working backward again until they find the source of that person's illness (whether it's another person, or, at the end of the line, the bacterium, virus, or other cause).

When people are infected at roughly the same time, scientists can use genomic sequencing of the germ to determine what strain of a virus or bacterium a person is infected with and then trace its history back. In the case of the patient from Snohomish County, it didn't take long for doctors to put two and two together and realize that the patient must have become infected in Wuhan while visiting family and returned to the US before he had begun to exhibit symptoms. But was he the first US citizen to develop COVID-19? That wouldn't be known until months later.

Genomic Sequencing Is Not Just for People

One of the best tools that scientists have today to fight infectious disease is genomic sequencing. After all, until you know exactly what you're up against, it's hard to mount a successful defense. Sequencing the genome of germs is not a new technique, and it's how we know that the virus responsible for COVID-19 is a coronavirus, how to test if someone is infected, and for many pathogens, what the animal reservoir (the animal that the pathogen can live in) is—and when the disease first jumped into humans.

Scientists were already working on sequencing the SARS-CoV-2 viral genome as the first cases of a mysterious respiratory illness in Wuhan, China, were reported by the media. While scientists often toil away in relative isolation, public health work, by its very nature, is cooperative. On January 9, 2020, almost a week after the first reports of the virus reached the US, Chinese scientists shared the sequence of the virus's genome. The viral sequence told researchers a lot about the virus: it was newly discovered (novel), and it was a coronavirus in the same family as the viruses that cause MERS and SARS. Once the sequence of the virus was known, work could begin to develop the diagnostic tests, and ultimately the vaccines and treatments, that doctors could use on suspected patients.

Scientists can also use computational methods to trace back the lineage of a bacterial or viral infection, in much the same way you can go on any number of

genealogical websites to trace your family tree with DNA.
Genetic material tends to mutate at a certain rate—and in
some places, rarely or if ever at all. So, it can be used like a
molecular clock to tell scientists how "old" the genome of
something is. In the case of the SARS-CoV-2 pandemic,
many people started to wonder if they were actually
infected with COVID-19 in December or January—before
any cases had been identified in the US. Because many
respiratory viruses and bacteria can cause similar
symptoms, figuring out exactly what the cause of
someone's illness is relies on this kind of molecular testing.

Remember that the sequence of genetic material is
like the blueprint for an organism (from a tiny bacterium
all the way to the largest mammal). Sections of the genome
correspond to genes, which in turn result in proteins that
create molecules. If a molecule is essential for life, it's not
likely that section of the genome will change very much.
This is the reason why genetic mutations in some genes can
have such devastating consequences, such as a shortened
lifespan, to those who are affected. But there are other
sections of the genome that can change without very much
of an impact to the individual. The same way that humans
have different eye or hair colors, other organisms can have
slightly different characteristics that don't negatively
impact their ability to survive. And some changes that
occur might give the organism an advantage over others:
think of insects or plants that give off an unpleasant taste
that keeps them from being eaten. Using this molecular
clock of mutation rates, scientists gain insight into how a
germ's genome changed over time and spread through a
population.

To learn if the SARS-CoV-2 virus had been
circulating around the US before the outbreak in
Washington put the nation on alert, scientists looked for a
signature of the virus in a material that would have been
routinely collected from otherwise healthy people in
December 2019 and early January 2020—donated blood.
In leftover samples from blood donated between

December 13, 2019, and January 17, 2020, researchers looked for antibodies to SARS-CoV-2 using a variety of methods. In more than seven thousand samples from donors in nine states (California, Connecticut, Iowa, Massachusetts, Michigan, Oregon, Rhode Island, Washington, and Wisconsin), 106 were broadly reactive, and eighty-four had neutralizing activity. These findings mean it was likely that SARS-CoV-2, the virus that causes COVID-19, was in the US weeks before the first cases were identified—and was already spreading across the country. With what we now know about asymptomatic COVID-19 infections, and how many people have only mild symptoms, like a runny nose or slight cough (symptoms that are pretty general and mimic the common cold and allergies), finding Patient Zero for this pandemic may be next to impossible.

From Sequence to Treatment to Vaccine

Once the genetic sequence of the virus was learned, researchers around the world began work to develop a test for it. Before genetic sequencing, it could take a long time for doctors to pinpoint the bacteria or virus causing infection: the likely organism had to be isolated and multiplied to a sufficient number to allow for testing, and then sometimes multiple tests had to be performed to identify exactly what it was. It could take a few days to a week or more for some bacteria to grow enough—be "cultured"—and that's assuming the ideal growth conditions (temperature, light, and surface/food for the organism). Even after correctly identifying the microorganism, there could still be other tests to figure out what medications it is susceptible to.

If a person has an infection, it's important to learn exactly what is causing it so that the right antibiotic or other medication can be given—before the infection gets out of control—making rapid diagnostic tests highly desirable.

There are a number of different methods that scientists have at their disposal to identify an infectious organism.

One is the polymerase chain reaction (PCR). PCR works by making many copies of specific regions of the organism's genome (amplifying it), greatly speeding up the time it takes to have enough parts to identify the bacteria or virus. You don't need the entire genome of the organism either—you can target specific sections that are unique, and some PCR methods let you look for multiple organisms at once. Importantly, each PCR cycle takes only minutes, and most can be completed in an hour or less! This is a tremendous advantage over the slow-growing culture methods, where identifying more than one pathogen at the same time can be difficult.

With PCR testing available, doctors could compare patient samples to the known sequence of the coronavirus, differentiating between those who had just a cold or the flu and patients who had the novel COVID-19. Developing accurate diagnostics tests is only one benefit of genomic sequencing, as I'll explain next.

AI and Machine Learning to the Rescue: Drug Repurposing and Vaccine Development

In Chapter Seven, we saw that it can take a decade or more and a few billion dollars to bring a new drug on the market. In that chapter, I explained that AI and machine learning are cutting that timeline down, substantially in some cases, by using computers to play out scenarios that predict how well a drug will work and reduce the number of dead-end molecules that would otherwise have to be tested. A simple way to think about this is to imagine a video game where your goal is to match the right key into the lock—but you have hundreds or thousands or even millions of keys to test. Each is ever so slightly different, and maybe multiple keys will fit, but only one or a small few will actually open the lock. As you move through the game, you might figure out that you can eliminate a bunch of keys if they aren't the right shape. In this analogy, the lock is the target, and the keys are the different molecules that need testing. These methods aren't just used for new drugs—they can also be used on existing drugs to find new purposes for them. Repurposing existing drugs for a new indication can dramatically speed up the approval process; after all, the drugs have already been shown to be safe in humans, and they have already undergone clinical trials for a different need. In 2020, scientists were doing just this to find treatments for COVID-19.

Once scientists identified that the organism causing COVID-19 was a virus, it made sense to identify antiviral medications that might work to stop the infection, and several showed promise. Researchers used AI techniques to find potential antiviral drugs that were known to work against viruses that were similar genetically to SARS-CoV-2. Scanning through the vast amount of scientific literature to find proverbial needles in the haystack is one of the things AI can do much more efficiently than humans. Remdesivir is a drug that works by stopping the virus from making copies of its genome—effectively stopping the virus in its tracks. Initially targeted to work against the virus that causes Ebola, remdesivir was granted emergency use by the FDA for patients with COVID-19 on May 1, 2020. Other antiviral medications tested against COVID-19 included lopinavir, ritonavir (both approved for HIV), danoprevir (Hepatitis C), and favipiravir (influenza).

Researchers around the world screened almost twelve thousand drug compounds in a drug "library" from Scripps Research Institute in California for COVID-19 treatment effectiveness. They identified twenty-one molecules, including remdesivir, that stopped SARS-CoV-2 infected cells from growing. Apilimod, a drug investigated for use in autoimmune conditions such as Crohn's disease and rheumatoid arthritis, and clofazimine, which treats leprosy, are among the most promising candidates based on this early study.' Clinical trials for these drugs and others repurposed for COVID-19 are ongoing, but the speed at which they were identified remains impressive—and due in large part to computational strategies used to identify them.

Existing drugs are just one avenue of research scientists can pursue during a pandemic. The same AI and machine learning techniques to develop new drugs that I described in Chapter Seven more generally can be used in a public health crisis like a disease outbreak too. Once researchers know the genetic makeup of the organism, they can design new molecules to target specific areas, like the proteins that help the virus or bacteria enter our cells, evade our natural immune system defenses, or make them susceptible to specific treatments. It can also be used to design vaccines that teach our immune system what the germ looks like before we are infected, helping us stop the infection before it can even start.

Vaccines at the Speed of Light

Never before has the scientific community rallied around a cause as rapidly as it did to create not just one, but several, vaccines in roughly twelve months from the time the outbreak first started. While there is no doubt that the organized effort and infusion of funding helped, everything I've described in this chapter was made possible by AI, machine learning, and big data.

Much of the success for vaccine development is a result of knowing the genomic sequence of the virus as rapidly as we did. As I described, once you have that information, you can design a vaccine that can prime our immune system against specific characteristics of the pathogen. It can be highly specific and give you immunity to only a single strain of an organism (this is a bit like the flu vaccine—where scientists target what they think the dominant strains during a particular flu season will be) or more general, where you'd be protected against multiple strains or similar organisms.

But even knowing the specific genomic sequence isn't always enough—after all, we don't have durable vaccines yet for a number of diseases and illnesses, like the common cold or HIV. Some viruses have a particularly insidious weapon called "viral escape" (see "Shutdowns, Quarantines, and 'Flattening the Curve': The Language of Pandemics" below) and change substantially enough so that our immune systems fail to recognize it and can't mount the appropriate immune response. This is where machine learning and AI can help.

Through computational modeling, which simulates how something might occur, scientists can predict how an organism might mutate based on its past behavior and design vaccines that account for those potential mutations. For example, one strain of a virus might mutate in precisely the same spot after it comes into contact with a strain from another part of the world or one that developed in a different organism, like a bat or a bird—something that could easily happen as a virus spreads through a population. They can even match specific mutations or strains to geographic regions (Figure 8.2). If you think about your immune system like a large building with thousands of locked doors, each germ (and all of its possible permutations) is a key and fits exactly one lock. So, we can design a vaccine to precisely match one door, which puts us at a disadvantage if the pathogen mutates, or we can use modeling to design one that works in multiple doors—like a master key to the entire building.

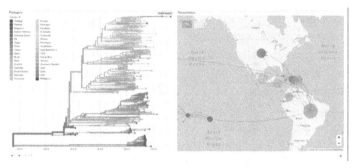

Figure 8.2. Computational modeling showing the different strains of
bacteria and their relationship to geographic location.
[https://pubmed.ncbi.nlm.nih.gov/30135232/]

What's more, researchers who are part of
Harvard's Human Immunomics Initiative are also using AI
to model the best ways to activate our immune systems and
to learn how people who are vaccinated might respond.
Because our immune system changes as we age, it's
important to consider when the best time to be vaccinated
might be—something that would otherwise take decades
to figure out. AI can help us rapidly sift through millions,
billions, even trillions of scenarios, giving scientists a
handful of promising options to test.

Sidebar:
Are We Ready for AI-driven Vaccine Development?

It's one thing to be able to go from outbreak to
vaccine in a little more than a year, it's quite another to do
it over and over again. In Chapter Seven, I wrote about the
very long, expensive road from hopeful molecule to FDA-
approved and on-the-market drug: a timeframe of more
than a decade and more than a billion dollars is not
uncommon. But I also described how AI and machine
learning are helping scientists to get a jump start on that
process, using the technologies to (virtually) sift through
thousands of candidates in a fraction of the time it would
take someone at the lab bench. And they are being used to
find new applications for existing drugs. The example of

antivirals for Hepatitis C or leprosy drugs being tested in COVID-19 patients are just a few examples. The road to developing a vaccine is no less complicated or short.

Vaccine (and drug) development today looks quite different from fifty or even twenty years ago. From computationally modeling the medication or vaccine and its interactions with both our immune system and the pathogen, to virtual clinical trials with remote monitoring and complex computational studies, that protracted timeline keeps getting shorter and shorter. Yet even though scientists cheer the reduction in time to bring helpful—sometimes lifesaving—drugs to patients, there can be uncertainty and wariness by the average person about these rapidly approved medications.

One of the most common reasons for refusing any of the COVID-19 vaccines was concern that they had been developed too quickly and not adequately tested. A study found that among those responding that they would not pursue getting vaccinated against COVID-19, nearly 18 percent indicated they felt the vaccine wouldn't be safe, and more than 15 percent said they didn't think the vaccine would be effective. A poll by the Kaiser Family Foundation in December 2020 found that more than 20 percent of those responding felt the vaccine development process was moving too quickly.

As researchers integrate machine learning and AI into the drug and vaccine development pipeline, that decade or longer timeframe is going to get shorter and shorter. In order to maintain the public's trust in vaccines, scientists are going to have to get better at explaining how they aren't cutting corners in development—they're taking advantage of a technology that lets them get lifesaving vaccines in arms faster by speeding up the preclinical processes and letting machine learning help find the best candidate drugs to test (Figure 8.3). They're using computers to model thousands or even millions of different ways a particular vaccine or drug might interact with common medications someone could be taking, so that researchers can know, before a patient ever takes the actual drug, whether or not a drug interaction (and the negative outcomes associated with that) will happen— particularly as pharmaceutical companies turn to new methods of making vaccines, like mRNA, which can be scaled up more quickly than traditional methods and don't involve using weakened (attenuated) or inactivated versions of the germ.

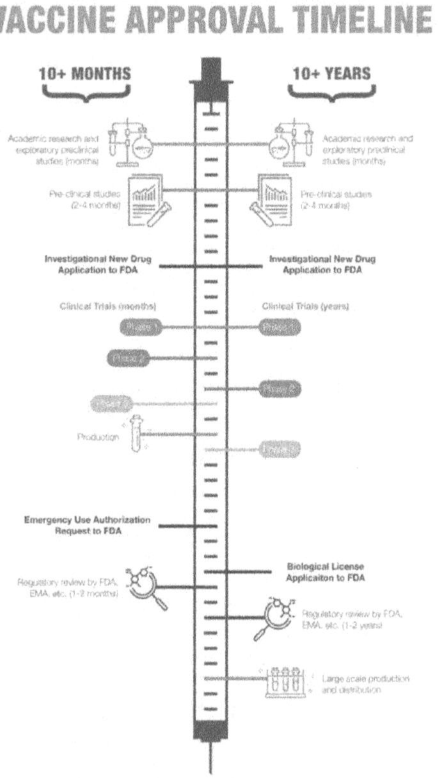

Figure 8.3. Rapid vaccine development compared to standard timeline. [https://tristatehospital.org/covid-19-vaccine-approval-timeline/].

What's more, the extensive modeling the new vaccines and drugs will undergo before clinical trials means that they can be more effective and with fewer side effects than existing options. Scientists will better predict which patients are likely to have the best response to a vaccine, what side effects will develop and in which patients, and how often you'll need to be vaccinated—before the vaccine even gets into human trials. We may even see a time where we have personalized vaccines, designed specifically for you, that take into account your existing health, any chronic illnesses you might have, and medications you take.

In this new age of machine learning and AI, we'll all have to rethink (and relearn) what we know about vaccine development. When an outbreak happens, the ability to repurpose existing drugs and create a new vaccine at light speed will be crucial to save lives.

Shutdowns, Quarantines, and "Flattening The Curve": The Language of Pandemics

I've joked that we all became armchair epidemiologists in 2020 because of COVID-19, but the reality is that the pandemic forced us to learn, or at least become used to hearing, terminology that generally only scientists and researchers were comfortable with. Raise your hand if you know what R_0 or PCR are. (Don't worry—there's no multiple-choice quiz to come.) If you're unclear about some of the terms I've used in this chapter or that you've heard on the news, these definitions might be helpful.

Antibody: a protein made by our immune system in response to an antigen. We produce antibodies after direct exposure or after vaccination, and they can neutralize the foreign antigen.

Antigen: a substance that causes the immune system to produce antibodies or have some kind of response. Toxins made by some kinds of bacteria, proteins on the outside of bacteria or viruses, and pollen from grasses and trees are examples.

Attenuated vaccines: vaccines made with a weakened living version of the germ that is not infectious but will still activate the immune system and production of antibodies. The measles-mumps-rubella (MMR) vaccine is an example of an attenuated vaccine.

Case Fatality Rate (CFR): measures the proportion of deaths in people who have been diagnosed with a condition. A disease with a CFR=0 doesn't cause any deaths, while one with a CFR=100 percent kills everyone. The 1918 Spanish influenza pandemic had a CFR≈2.5 percent, while the 2013-2016 Ebola epidemic had a CFR of 89.1 percent in Sierra Leone. Most flu pandemics have a CFR<0.1 percent.

Coronaviruses: a family of viruses that can be identified by a distinguishing crown ("corona") of spiky proteins on its surface. These viruses cause disease in both humans and animals and can have respiratory, gastrointestinal, or neurologic symptoms.

COVID-19: the disease caused by the SARS-CoV-2 virus. The "-19" reflects that it was discovered in 2019.

Epidemiology: the study of health and disease conditions in populations. Infectious disease and public health are key aspects of epidemiology.

"Flattening the curve": a phrase that was widely used during the COVID-19 pandemic to demonstrate how quarantines, shelter-in-place rules, and closing of businesses and schools could prevent health systems from being overwhelmed with patients.

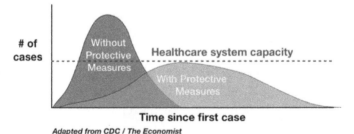

Adapted from CDC / The Economist

Figure 8.4. Healthcare system capacity.
(https://www.nytimes.com/article/flatten-curve-coronavirus.html)

Infectivity: the ability of a germ to infect a person or animal.

Live vaccines: vaccines produced with weakened forms of the virus (attenuated). They are still "alive," but because of attenuation, they will not cause illness in someone with a healthy immune system.

MERS (Middle East Respiratory Syndrome): MERS is caused by the MERS coronavirus and was the source of outbreaks in 2012 and 2018 in Saudi Arabia and 2015 in South Korea. Symptoms of MERS include fever, cough, shortness of breath, and gastrointestinal upset.

Mode of transmission for a pathogen: it can be ingested (eaten), inhaled (breathed in), or can spread through direct contact (like sexually transmitted diseases) or by a vector (insects like mosquitoes, ticks, or rats).

mRNA vaccines: they work by getting our cells to make a harmless protein (antigen), causing an immune response like the building up of antibodies, so that our immune system will recognize the pathogen if it tries to infect us later.

Outbreak (Not just the 1995 film depicting the spread of an Ebola-like virus in the US): an outbreak is an increase from the normal baseline of disease in a specific geographic region.

Pandemic: an outbreak that has spread across an entire country, continent, or the world.

Pathogen: any microorganism that can cause disease. Even seemingly harmless bacteria and viruses can become pathogenic.

Polymerase chain reaction (PCR): a molecular biology technique that is used to create many copies of specific regions of the genome. It has many applications, including identifying if a person has been infected with a pathogen.

R_0 *or "R naught"*: a way to describe how infectious a disease is by calculating the number of additional people each person who has the disease can infect.

Reservoir: the organism that a pathogenic microorganism can live in and multiple/carry out its life cycle. The reservoir does not normally become ill but can inadvertently pass the pathogen on to another animal or to humans.

SARS: Severe Acute Respiratory Syndrome caused by the SARS-coronavirus (SARS-CoV-1). Symptoms of SARS are similar to that of the flu: fever, sore throat, cough, muscle pain, and extreme tiredness. Diarrhea is common with SARS, as are shortness of breath and pneumonia in more severe cases. SARS was the cause of an outbreak from 2002–2004 that involved twenty-nine countries, affected more than eight thousand people, and led to the deaths of more than 770 people worldwide.

SARS-CoV-2: the virus that causes the COVID-19 disease. Its full name is the severe acute respiratory syndrome (SARS) coronavirus 2 (CoV-2).

Spike proteins: the protein molecules that are on the surface of the SARS-CoV-2 virus and are a target of mRNA vaccination.

Vaccination: a method of exposing the immune system to a pathogen in order to prevent (serious) infection exposed later.

Viral escape: occurs when an organism's genomic mutations change it enough that the infected host's immune system no longer recognizes the pathogen, even if previously vaccinated.

Virulence: a measurement of how serious or harmful a disease is.

—End Sidebar—

The Future You: Pandemic-prepared

In this chapter, I've tried to give you some perspective about the COVID-19 pandemic and our response to it. More importantly, it gives you a sneak peek into how we can be ready for the next pandemic. Here's what that could look like:

- We'll be using AI-enabled platforms to continuously monitor global conditions, so we have a heads up about the next pandemic—before it starts. BlueDot, a Canadian company launched in 2014, scans news around the world (in more than sixty languages) and reports on animal disease outbreaks and airline data to identify potential outbreaks as they happen. Its machine learning and natural language processing methods filter through hundreds of local news reports, looking for evidence of illness that could potentially lead to an outbreak. This allowed it to warn its customers on December 31, 2019—a full week before the CDC and ten days before the World Health Organization.

- The global surveillance for potential outbreaks will make it easier for public health officials to identify the first patients with the disease. Identifying those individuals and then using epidemiology and old-fashioned detective work, doctors may be able to isolate and treat them before they can infect others—possibly halting the next pandemic in its tracks.

- Our personal devices (smartphones, fitness/sleep trackers, smartwatches, and more) will let us know if the sniffles and slight cough we have are actually allergies, a simple cold, or something worse, and can help doctors remotely monitor our health status. The most recent version of the Apple Watch, for example, can measure blood oxygen levels—a key measurement for how well someone is breathing—and heart rate. And the Warrior Watch study of healthcare workers from Mount Sinai Health System in New York found that longitudinal heart rate variability data combined with surveys were able to predict COVID-19 diagnosis. There'll be greater interest in using this data to pinpoint with greater accuracy where micro-outbreaks are happening, in real time. In large cities, this could mean one city block at a time, giving doctors in those areas a heads up about a potential influx of patients and giving the general population enough warning to avoid certain places until the crisis has passed.

- Scientists will identify the causes of new outbreaks at even faster speeds. Genomic sequencing has already moved from expensive novelty technology available at only the most advanced academic medical centers to relatively cheap and almost commonplace usage around the world. And sequencing won't just help us to label the germ, it'll give us a leg up on figuring out how to treat it— and prevent it with new vaccines.

- Equipment and goods shortages, like we all saw at the beginning of the COVID-19 pandemic, won't be as severe—if they happen at all. By coordinating the transportation and manufacturing needs with the outbreak and pandemic spread, we'll be able to avoid running out of PPE, hand sanitizer, or toilet paper. When shipping and factories are at risk in certain regions due to increased illness, robots and drones can help pack boxes and make sure home delivery isn't disrupted.

- We'll be able to respond to natural disasters like devastating hurricanes, floods, and earthquakes better. Lessons learned from the COVID-19 pandemic go far beyond infectious disease, and outbreaks often go hand in hand with natural disasters due to disruptions of existing systems to keep them in check. We can expect to see governments and other organizations use AI and machine learning strategies to model and prepare for the next disaster.

- The rapid pace of COVID-19 vaccine development isn't likely to go away. While we may not see new vaccines or medications come on the market in less than a year, like we saw with COVID-19, without the same global motivations and influx of money, there's little incentive across all stakeholders to go back to the decade-long system. AI and machine learning are directly responsible for helping research move at this frantic pace, but questions remain about whether the average person will accept these drugs and vaccines without understanding how and why they can be developed so quickly.

- A cure for the common cold? New methods of vaccine development, such as mRNA technology, may finally give scientists the key to creating a universal cold or flu vaccine. No longer tied to using weakened or dead pathogens to make vaccines, scientists have leveraged the power of genomics to teach our immune systems. Other diseases, like HIV, might also see an effective vaccine using these methods.

Are You Ready for the Future?

While we all hope that the next pandemic is decades (or longer) away, there are things we can do now to be prepared:

1. Connected devices, smartwatches, and smartphone apps are great for helping us track our sleep, fitness, and other health measurements. In an outbreak, they can help you know when you should contact the doctor or seek immediate emergency care and monitor your vital signs.
2. Connected devices are also proving their worth by helping to predict whether you might have COVID-19 before any symptoms develop. The Oura Ring and Apple Watch, for example, both predicted positive COVID-19 tests—days before the users felt ill. If your watch or other wearable could alert you to the possibility you might be sick, you'd have the opportunity to change your

behaviors, get tested earlier, and stock up on chicken noodle soup.

3. Worried that the COVID-19 vaccines were rushed because of the pandemic? Just knowing how AI and machine learning are transforming drug and vaccine development and clinical trials can help you avoid falling prey to rumors that new drugs or vaccines aren't tested thoroughly or aren't effective.

CHAPTER NINE:

THE CONCERNS, HURDLES, AND HARMS OF SMART MEDICINE

"Man is still the most extraordinary computer of all." —John F. Kennedy

AI will change medicine in incredible ways, empowering patients to take control of their health while increasing the quality of care and helping doctors better prevent and treat disease. Yet alongside these advantages will come considerable drawbacks, as AI promises to disrupt medicine, threaten patient privacy, and raise ethical questions about what machines can and should be allowed to do.

For example, if expecting parents can edit a gene for a rare disease in their unborn babies, should they also be able to edit other genes for eye color, athletic propensity, or creative talent? If AI can predict a patient will die within a year, should physicians still prioritize their care in areas where hospitals are overcrowded and understaffed? If you have the ability to find out the genetic defects you possess, would you want to know, even if there was nothing doctors could do? And what if the technology makes an inaccurate prediction? With how quickly the science is moving, what's inaccurate or incomplete today may not be in the near future.

Not surprisingly, many doctors and patients are resistant to using smart machines in medicine, even if their hospitals and medical centers are already using AI and machine learning algorithms to spot at-risk patients. Many argue quality healthcare requires compassion, something computers don't possess. This begs the question of how big of a role AI should have in our health. What kind of care should we allow computers to give? Which medical decisions should be made by doctors and which made by machines? And what happens if scientists learn how to program computers to show compassion and other human emotions?

AI's adoption in healthcare will also threaten jobs—though not likely those of healthcare professionals whose position entails the kind of direct patient interaction that can't be easily transferred to a machine. Though it may result in the elimination of some jobs altogether, they will most likely be the kinds of tasks that lend themselves to automation, while creating new opportunities, especially for computer and data specialists. And we will need people who can act as the interface between the patient and the computer—folks who have some level of specialized medical and scientific training, and who are fantastic at conveying the human touch when it's needed.

The technology will change how doctors and other healthcare practitioners are trained. Even though most medical schools today provide little to no preparation on data-driven software or other computerized tools, medical education has already evolved to encompass training in electronic health records, and some have called for a revamp of physician curriculum and training to include working with and managing AI systems. Virtual and augmented reality are giving hopeful doctors and nurses a chance to practice their skills on virtual patients, over and over and in the face of any kind of complication the computer can simulate. That kind of experience will give students who use those tools the advantage when they encounter actual patients. Still, changes to how future doctors are trained are likely to occur somewhat organically in the years to come, as medical schools will broaden what their students know in order to remain competitive.

Finally, privacy and security concerns will continue to haunt AI in healthcare. Many patients are already uncomfortable with the idea that their health data is being shared whenever they use smartphone apps, wearable sensors, and electronic health records, even if their anonymity is preserved. If you've been to the doctor or hospital in the past few years, you've probably been asked to sign a consent form allowing researchers to use your data—often stripped of the identifying information that could point it back to you. And you may be asked to consent to varying levels of data access. For example, allowing researchers to use any leftover blood that was taken for routine lab work to be used for population-level genetic testing or letting doctors access your medical record to determine if you're eligible for a research study.

Others worry what will happen if hackers access large patient databanks or AI-enabled medical machines. It's one thing to have an outage of a system that takes AI prediction down; after all, doctors have the necessary training to give their patients a prognosis without AI. AI is just making that process more efficient and often more accurate. But it's completely another to have hackers able to change the settings remotely of equipment that runs the AI software. For example, pacemaker settings hacked to deliver lethal jolts or reprogrammed not to work when they are supposed to. Researchers at the University of Alabama even demonstrated that they could change the settings on a mannequin used for medical student training, suggesting that other connected devices could be at risk in a hospital setting. With data breaches already costing hospitals millions of dollars annually, there's tremendous pressure on the technology side to fix the existing problems and prepare organizations for what's to come.

In this chapter, I'll give you a peek into the dark side of all this technology and how it could impact health and wellness. While we don't have to worry (at least not yet) about robots taking over our lives (and health), it's common sense to at least know of, if not understand, some of the downfalls of relying on these new technologies. I'll start with some of the ethical issues that have been raised and then describe the technical challenges with all this data before hitting on some of the privacy concerns. The ideas in this chapter aren't meant to make you turn into a tech-phobic person anxious to return to the pre-Internet/AI/technology era—after all, nearly all of the problems and potential downfalls I'll describe in the pages to come are being tackled by experts today. But I hope it will help you to understand what the challenges are, and how you can use that information to make more informed decisions.

The Ethical Dilemma: Just Because We Can Do It Doesn't Mean We Should

The questions about the ethics of using AI and machine learning technologies in healthcare aren't dissimilar to worries posed for any new technology in virtually every industry—healthcare and wellness aren't unique. Over time as new technologies move from novelties with few users to nearly ubiquitous (think about the adoption of smartphones), we see that some of the initial worries never came to pass, or solutions were found, and other challenges we didn't even think of have become real problems. Let's unpack some of the issues facing AI and machine learning.

As I described in Chapter Five (Unlocking the Language of Life), machine learning and AI are helping doctors and researchers move gene editing from sci-fi fantasy to real-world patients. CRISPR is curing sickle cell anemia and beta thalassemia, related diseases that are significantly disabling to those who have them, and there is real interest in using similar gene-editing techniques to cure all sorts of devastating conditions like Huntington's disease or chronic conditions like multiple sclerosis.

If you're like most Americans, you probably agree with the results of a 2018 poll by the Associated Press–NORC (National Opinion Research) Center for Public Affairs Research at the University of Chicago that curing people of devastating diseases like Huntington's are excellent uses of gene-editing technology, and something you'd support. But where do we draw the line? Do you feel differently about using gene editing in an adult to treat a disorder they have already been diagnosed with versus one that they will develop, but don't have any evidence of? What about changing an adult's genome to fix a genetic mutation that only makes it more likely someone will develop a disorder—where it's not 100 percent guaranteed?

These are some of the thornier issues that both doctors/scientists and society have to grapple with in the upcoming years. Where do we stand on gene editing for *BRCA1/2* mutations, for example? Although the risks of developing breast or ovarian cancer by age eighty are roughly 70 percent for mutations in either gene, it's not guaranteed that a mutation will definitely lead to cancer for any one individual. What about some of the other genes that are associated with a higher risk of developing cancer, but not as high a risk as *BRCA1/2*? Would you support gene editing in those situations? And at what age would you have someone undergo CRISPR treatment? Would you wait until they are thirty? Twenty? Or would you want them to have it done when they are a child? What about having it done when a couple undergoes assistive reproductive techniques, like in vitro fertilization (IVF)?

These are complicated ethical questions that society has been grappling with for years—decades, in some cases—even before you throw in the complexities of AI. What AI can do is help us to work through complex models, showing us every possible outcome and the probability it will occur. And the answers to some of the challenges might not look very different from the solutions we've already come up with for other technologies. For example, in response to the backlash over the data companies were getting from us each time we visited a website, users now can decide whether or not the website can store cookies on our computer or share our information with other companies.

The answers to these questions might be different when we think about noncancer diseases or conditions that aren't necessarily debilitating. Inherited deafness is a common disability, affecting approximately one in every

one thousand newborns, and nearly one hundred genes
have been associated with deafness. There has been
interest in using gene-editing techniques to restore hearing
in patients whose hearing loss is caused by a genetic
mutation, and they've proven successful in mouse
experiments. The "Beethoven" mutation, named for the
famous deaf composer, causes progressive hearing loss
that leaves people deaf by their mid-twenties. In an
experiment at Harvard Medical School and Boston
Children's Hospital, scientists used CRISPR to edit the
"Beethoven" mutation in mice, enabling the mice to
maintain the ability to hear throughout their lives, and
giving hope that a similar cure could be on the horizon for
human patients.

Still, not everyone is happy about the scientific
advances and the potential to cure deafness (or other
disabilities) in humans. Deaf culture advocates and others
are concerned about the "erasure" of people with
disabilities in society: using CRISPR and other gene-editing
technologies to "fix" a trait, ultimately leading to fewer
individuals with that condition, potentially making it more
difficult for their needs to be met and exacerbating social
and medical inequalities. Among parents of children with
Down syndrome, a genetic condition caused by an extra
copy of the twenty-first chromosome (trisomy 21), there
are a range of opinions. Even the word "disability"
suggests something that needs to be fixed or made normal,
a viewpoint that many researchers in the field as well as
parents and patient advocacy groups bristle against. And
the idea of using CRISPR or similar techniques to create
"designer babies"—children whose eye or hair color,
athletic prowess, or intellectual abilities could be ordered
on demand—seemed like the line that scientists (and
society) were unwilling to cross.

Until 2018, these ethical questions appeared to be
little more than a thought exercise without real-world
application. That changed when a scientist from China
announced he had used CRISPR in human embryos from

IVF, and that one woman had given birth to twin girls. The scientist's plan was to use the gene-editing technique to alter a gene called CCR5, with the goal of making the resulting babies resistant to diseases like HIV, smallpox, and cholera—diseases that, with the exception of smallpox, which was eradicated in 1980, remain the cause of significant disease around the world. Though scientists and governments around the world soundly rebuked the Chinese man for his work, a Pandora's box has been opened, and it's unclear how far we're willing to take it.

What's more, scientists still don't know the long-term consequences of altering *every* nucleotide of our DNA. Where one change could prevent breast cancer, would it also make someone more likely to have autism or bipolar disorder, become blind in their fifties, or predispose the person to dementia when he or she turns seventy-five? Not every change would necessarily be "bad," but it might depend on where the person lived or the environmental exposures the person came into contact with. For example, the same genetic mutation that causes sickle cell anemia (see Chapter Five) and causes red blood cells to be sickle-shaped also makes someone less prone to malaria. So, if you lived in a country where your risk of malaria was very high, you might not want to CRISPR away your genetic mutation.

One of the ways researchers use machine learning is for predictive analytics, as I've explained in several of the previous chapters. These can be anything from predicting who is likely to develop diabetes among individuals with a slightly high BMI but normal glucose test to which patients in an ICU will die from sepsis. (Spoiler: doctors already use these sepsis-spotting algorithms at hospitals across the country and around the world to identify these at-risk patients—this isn't just a hypothetical scenario.)

Imagine a hospital with a single empty bed left and two patients who need to be admitted. Who should doctors choose, and who should they turn away? Consider an epidemic where a limited amount of a potentially lifesaving drug is available and twice as many people need it. (COVID-19 may come to mind.) No matter what we might think or hope about healthcare, there is a limited amount of resources, be it hospital or ICU beds or medications, and some amount of rationing is inevitable. What might happen when an AI program or machine learning algorithm predicts that one of the patients in the above scenario is ten times more likely to die than the other patient—even with medical intervention? Should doctors prioritize the healthier individual?

This is another one of those ethical dilemmas facing doctors today. As AI and machine learning simultaneously improve healthcare by helping clinicians diagnose cancer a year or more before they'd get picked up through normal methods, the technologies are causing some worry about exacerbating health disparities. The old adage, "Garbage in, garbage out," applies, especially for AI and machine learning algorithms. If the data used to train the system is flawed in the first place, through missing data that emphasizes one patient group over another, or fails to include enough persons of non-White ancestry, for example, to be representative of the general population, the resulting prediction model could also be flawed and lead to inappropriate actions. What we need to do is use the power of AI to keep one or more of those sick patients from reaching the hospital in the first place. If you know you're at risk for a particular illness when there's still time to prevent it or at least minimize its effects, some of those ethical dilemmas might disappear entirely.

Algorithms built in response to COVID-19 to help hospitals decide which patients to put on ventilators or who to send to the ICU were called into question for exactly this problem. A review of models used to predict the diagnosis or prognosis of COVID-19 infections found that *all* included algorithms had a high risk of bias. Even before the recent pandemic, researchers comparing who was targeted for participation in a program for patients with complex health needs found the algorithm predicted healthcare costs—not health conditions—and was racially biased.

The good news: we can fix this problem. Scientists are working on methods to minimize and eliminate the biases that may be found in existing prediction models and determine best practices to prevent them from creeping into new algorithms when they are made. And they're also working on using AI proactively to reduce existing biases in healthcare. For example, patients with chronic pain are often labeled as "opioid-seeking," and their complaints are minimized by healthcare providers. Other patients may have their treatment determined by the level of pain they are in. If you're suffering from excruciating knee pain, your doctor might be more likely to recommend surgery than an anti-inflammatory drug. It's not hard to see how patients would be treated and the level of care they receive might be different based on whether or not the doctor believes how much the knee hurts.

Enter AI. Using deep learning, researchers trained systems to better match X-ray images to the level of pain a patient reported. Then they compared their model to the Kellgren-Lawrence Grade (KLG), the standard method to calculate pain levels from X-ray images. What the scientists found was that their model was more accurate at matching patient-reported pain levels than the KLG, especially for Black patients. Amazingly, it reduced the racial disparities by nearly half, compared to the KLG.

When the Machine Makes the Diagnosis

If you could have an expert doctor or an AI algorithm diagnose you, and both performed at the same level of accuracy (let's assume 85 percent for both), which would you choose? If you're like most people today, you'd probably choose the doctor. Now, what if the AI was better than the doctor, say close to 100 percent accuracy? Would you still choose the human? Chances are, you would. Or do you think it would depend on some factor, say how old you are or how comfortable you are with science and technology?

Researchers are starting to dig deeper into the reasons why this is the case. After all, AI algorithms have already been shown to out-diagnose even the best of doctors for some conditions and to identify potentially serious cancers earlier than their human counterparts. But there is still a lot of hesitation and resistance to using AI— for both doctors and patients. Researchers at New York University have found that one of the biggest factors is how we perceive ourselves.

As humans, we naturally understand ourselves to be unique. As a result, we sometimes carry that perception to include the things we do or how we experience what happens to us. If I get brain cancer, it's not just glioblastoma, it's my glioblastoma. If we go to the doctor, they will understand this because they are also human, where the computer will think of me as just another person with glioblastoma.

So, doctors are faced with a growing problem: how to integrate AI and machine learning into practice, because it's good for the patient, without the patient feeling like he or she is being treated as "just another _____." In some places, AI is already working behind the scenes to help doctors without patients knowing.

M Health Fairview is a partnership between the University of Minnesota, the University's Physician Network, and Fairview Health Services, which serves the greater Minneapolis-St. Paul region. In February 2019, M Health Fairview began using an AI system to help doctors decide when patients would be ready for discharge. The problem? None of the patients knew.

When you need a surgery or other procedure in the hospital, you usually undergo an informed consent process. Unless there are reasons why it can't be done (like what might happen in an emergency situation when you're unconscious), before you're wheeled back into the operating or procedure room, someone will come to your bedside with a clipboard or electronic tablet and make sure you understand what's going to happen and the potential risks involved. When it comes to doctors and hospitals using AI to help guide your treatment, that's not standard practice (yet).

This is one of the legal and ethical challenges facing widespread use of AI and machine learning, and there are few answers today. Should patients be told anytime their physician uses an AI software to help make a diagnosis? Should admissions paperwork include language and an explanation that AI might be used by some hospital departments to make decisions about the length of time they will spend in the hospital, or their care if they are at risk of developing a serious condition like sepsis? What's the difference between AI and any other analytical software that's already being used?

And what if the AI system gets it wrong—missing a critical cancer diagnosis, for example? How will a patient or the patient's family know if the AI system is to blame without transparency about where the technology is used and the ability to track down where in the process the system made a mistake? It's fairly unlikely that without FDA approval an AI system would be allowed to make healthcare decisions completely without human oversight, but it's still an interesting question.

You might remember the "black box" problem of AI and machine learning from back in Chapter Five. As I wrote in that chapter, there is an effort underway to make the AI less opaque—optimally removing the "black box" nature of these software programs entirely. But today, it's unlikely that the doctor or hospital will be able to tell a patient exactly how that system works—just that it does.

Some of this goes back to what I said at the very beginning of this book: doctors and scientists might as well be speaking a completely different language than the rest of us when they talk about AI and other technologies. It's no wonder that patients (and even some physicians) struggle to understand the nuances of these programs.

This disconnect and failure to describe in easy-to-comprehend language what's happening with AI, even generally, leaves patients worried about these systems. What's more, most patients aren't in a position to ask their doctor directly if and how they are being used—they simply don't even know it's a possibility. That's why it's critical to empower patients, to bring them into the conversation by describing this technology and how it can be used.

The Data Issue

The problems with AI and machine learning in healthcare don't end with ethical questions for philosophers and lawyers to debate. The problems with AI can start at the very beginning—with the data that are used to train or validate the models. Think of it this way: if you're going to cook an elaborate dinner, maybe with several new recipes from various sites, and you use expired and spoiled vegetables or meat, chances are that your dinner isn't going to go well. That's a bit like how it is for AI and machine learning algorithms. What are some of the problems that data can have?

1. Data can be past its prime. Imagine you moved to Atlanta or Raleigh or Houston, cities that have experienced tremendous population growth over recent decades, and you were trying to learn your way around—but the only map you could use was one that was drafted in 1980! You'd probably spend most of your time confused about roads that had been expanded or renamed, or new roads where there shouldn't be (according to your old map), and generally lost and frustrated. Now imagine that problem with healthcare.

   This can be a problem, especially when the criteria for a diagnosis have changed over time. Patients from ten years ago might have been considered to have a disorder that today could be a different disorder entirely, or they might even be thought of as not having the condition. Think this isn't likely? Think again. The definition of autism has evolved significantly since the 1960s and has contributed to the higher prevalence of the disorder today. Who has high blood pressure and should take medication? The answer today is more people than in early 2017, when the American Heart Association and American College of Cardiology changed the definition of what qualified as high blood pressure.

2. Data can be biased. We've all heard about the problems with AI and facial recognition being biased against some racial and ethnic groups—a problem that the tech industry is actively working to fix. In healthcare, the bias might be a result of who and what data are used to train the AI. For example, let's say you are a doctor at a community hospital in rural New Mexico, where over the past five years there's been an uptick in the number of deaths due to heart failure in your community. Your department is concerned that the hospital isn't identifying these patients earlier in their disease, when there could be an opportunity to treat them and extend their lives. To fix this problem, you want to install software that will identify which patients are at risk of having heart failure. You reach out to a former colleague, now at the Mayo Clinic, who lets you know of an add-on to the EHR system that will do exactly that. It sounds like it could be exactly what you're looking for, but the Mayo population that the machine learning algorithm was trained in is nothing like your community. Will it work as well for your hospital?

This is at the heart of one of the criticisms levied against technology stalwart IBM's Watson for Oncology. After Watson won the game show *Jeopardy!* in 2011, IBM turned the powerful system on healthcare—specifically cancer. IBM trained Watson for Oncology at one of the US's leading cancer institutions: Memorial Sloan Kettering Cancer Center. Although the company marketed the Watson product around the world, customers (hospitals and doctors) complained that the treatment results it recommended were biased toward ones that would be recommended at Memorial Sloan Kettering and didn't take into account regional or local differences.

3. Data can be missing. This shouldn't come as a surprise to anyone—but how missing data is handled can be a problem. And it's important to know why the data is missing in the first place. To begin, scientists need to know if the missing data is randomly missing but could be related to other data you do have, not missing at random, or missing completely randomly. The last option is different from the first, in that the missing data isn't in any way related to any other data that they do have.

    For example, let's say you have a survey of people and ask what their eye color is, how old they were when they started driving, and if they enjoy swimming. After you collect the information, you find that twenty-one people didn't respond to the swimming question, and thirteen people didn't reply with their age when they began driving. Whether or not someone enjoys swimming has absolutely nothing to do with the age someone begins to drive. Those data would be missing completely at random.

There are basically two ways of handling missing data: removing it or using a statistical method called imputation, which estimates what the missing data likely was. For data that is randomly missing or missing completely at random, imputation is OK—it can mean that scientists have a much larger set of information to work from when creating a machine learning algorithm or AI software. But if the data is *not* missing randomly, for instance sex and testosterone levels (females also produce testosterone—just at much lower levels than males), imputation probably isn't the best choice. However, removing data comes with a consequence too: doing so can introduce bias (if more females than males are missing testosterone levels, removing those females from the data set can lead to an inflated overall testosterone level). It can also reduce the size of the data used to train the AI and machine learning algorithms, making it less useful for a situation when the larger the data set, the better.

4. Data can be misanalyzed or simply analyzed differently. Scientists might use the wrong statistical analysis when training an AI or machine learning algorithm. This isn't to say that some data scientists are nefarious and set out to manipulate their results in their analysis. What I'm referring to is inadvertent use—like using imputation to handle missing data when the appropriate decision would have been to remove that patient from the data set entirely.

What is more likely to happen is that the data could be analyzed correctly in different ways, leading to differing results. Take, for instance, algorithms that have been created to identify patients with obesity. A hospital might want to reach out to patients who meet eligibility criteria for bariatric surgery or who could be interested in a weight-loss or exercise program. But the question of how to analyze the vast amount of data contained in EHRs can be overwhelming. Which data do you choose and what methods do you use?

The National NLP Clinical Challenges (N2C2) are a case in point. Formerly known as the Informatics for Integrating Biology & the Bedside (i2b2) challenge, each year, a data set of de-identified patient data from EHRs are released. In 2008, the challenge was to determine, solely from the data set, which patients had obesity, and if they had any other health conditions, like high blood pressure or diabetes. Thirty teams participated—each tackling the problem in a different way and with variable success. A patient labeled as having obesity using one method might be labeled as not having obesity using another. When the answer can be fairly certain—either someone has a disorder or they don't—the results from AI and machine learning can be compared to what a trained professional would determine based on going through someone's EHR. But the healthcare questions aren't always so simple (and sometimes determining if someone has a condition isn't simple either). Imagine trying to find the cause of an illness: you'd need to know both when patients were exposed and make sure it was within the right time period before they would be expected to develop symptoms. Or methods developed at different medical centers that work well for their population but don't do as well when another hospital tries to implement it. With competing AI and machine learning algorithms, it can be hard to say just which one's right.

The challenges with data aren't insurmountable, however. For example, instead of using data from only one hospital to train machine learning systems, there could be rules that require data from multiple centers be used, or that the resulting algorithm be restricted to use only in certain locations where the patients more closely match the ones used to train the system. More probable are groups of hospitals coming together to share data in a responsible way. Not only will this help with the bias issue, but it can also minimize missing data. After all, the better the data going in—the better it mirrors the actual patient population—the better the AI model coming out.

The Privacy Issues

Have you ever had your identity stolen or had someone nab your credit card and run up thousands of dollars in charges before your bank put a stop to it? In today's digital age, we hear of this happening all too frequently, with retailers like Target paying $18.5 million because of a data breach that affected forty-one million customers.

Retailers aren't the only companies affected by hackers. Medical record data theft is big business, with the average breach costing $7.1 million. Recent breaches included more than six hundred fifty thousand patients of Health Share of Oregon, six hundred forty thousand patients of the Florida Orthopaedic Institute, and the Blackbaud breach that impacted upwards of ten million patients across dozens of healthcare organizations. The Florida breach was the result of a ransomware attack, where patient records were "held ransom" for money. Although the Institute's administration was able to resecure its system, it was learned that patient information was potentially exposed and downloaded during the attack. Ransomware attacks are particularly insidious to a hospital, because they effectively shut personnel out of the EHR or other essential data, forcing hospitals to pay quickly in order to restore access.

Some attacks on healthcare records, however, are preventable. The Health Share of Oregon attack was the result of a laptop that had been stolen from a vendor of the organization, calling attention to insufficient internal security protocols. A phishing attack—where hackers mimic emails or attachments from reliable sites to spread malware or computer viruses—was the cause of a breach by BJC HealthCare, headquartered in St. Louis, Missouri, that affected nearly three hundred thousand patients. Three employees had fallen victim to the scam, allowing access to their email accounts and other sensitive data. The patient data leaked included such personal information as medications, health insurance data, and Social Security numbers.

It's not just our EHR data that's at risk. All the connected devices, our digital scales and home blood pressure cuffs, our smart thermostats and wireless security systems, are also at risk. As more health information is collected by these devices, like blood pressure monitors, oxygen sensors, or scales, or we allow data captured by one device, like a GPS-enabled fitness tracker, to be shared with another, our risks expand beyond just health records.

When we willingly or unknowingly share this information with companies, how well they keep the data secure is not always clear. Beyond hacking, this data is valuable as a commodity—meaning the companies you share it with can capitalize on being able to package it and resell it to other companies who might target advertising. Large amounts of data from these devices make it easier to both give you the service you demand and open you up to risk. It's not difficult to see how this could go awry: the security system data is hacked, and thieves find out when you're out of town by analyzing how frequently your doors open/close, and if there's a pattern to it. Combined with data from your smart thermostat, refrigerator, or water heater, it's not hard to imagine why this data is so valuable to cybercriminals. Oh—you've programmed your house to remain at a chilly 60 degrees in the middle of winter? You aren't adding anything to your shopping list? You turned the temperature down on your water heater? You must be away for a while.

But despite the risk, for the most part, the benefits outweigh the potential downsides. You can see who is at the door, unlock the door remotely for your child after school, even talk to delivery people who leave packages on your porch. Your home can be comfortable and more energy efficient, and you don't have to worry about forgetting a gallon of milk the next time you head to the grocery store. For personal devices, the upsides are even more appreciable. You can skip a trip to the doctor for a quick blood pressure reading or weigh-in, your smartwatch can alert you to potential heart troubles, and your fitness tracker can encourage you to hit your goals. The data we willingly give up makes our lives better.

The Future You: Participatory Patients

While this chapter has provided some counterbalance to the growing number of pundits saying AI is the next cure for everything, it's not meant to make you want to curl up in the corner with dread or decide to just ignore it all. The fact is AI and machine learning *are* incredibly useful tools that can have real, positive impacts on nearly every aspect of our lives—we all just need to be mindful of the pitfalls that are out there and know how to avoid them (where we can).

And one thing to keep in mind: as patients and consumers, we rarely need or want to know how everything works. I drive my car comfortable in the knowledge that people far smarter than I am have designed it to work consistently and safely get me from point A to point B. When the rare breakdown occurs or the check engine light comes on, I don't give myself a crash course in automotive repair; I take my car to the mechanic, who fixes it.

Healthcare and wellness aren't that different at their core. We go to the doctor to get a diagnosis because we know that the years of specialized training and education make the doctor far more qualified than I am to diagnose a weird skin rash or the reason why I'm tired all the time. If AI systems make them even better at their job, do I really need to know how it works? Or do I just want the most accurate, fastest diagnosis (along with the necessary treatment) to get me back to 100 percent? I'd argue the latter.

Do We Need Training on How to Be Patients in the Era of AI?

That's not to say we should stay ignorant of these technologies. And if you're reading this book, you're already the kind of person who wants to know a little bit more about what they can do for you. But as a population, we might need some help in learning how to be patients in the age of AI.

What do I mean? I don't mean that we all have to go to graduate school and get an MD or PhD just to have a conversation with our personal physicians. But I do think it's important to understand that the language of medicine is changing. EHRs (electronic health records) were virtually unheard of only two decades ago—now every doctors' office (or dentist, or veterinarian, or ...) has a medical records system. Logging onto your EHR to schedule an appointment or ask your doctor or nurse a question is commonplace. We're getting health and scientific news thrown at us from many angles—the recent COVID-19 pandemic is a case in point. When our local community papers start publishing articles about the differences between mRNA and attenuated vaccines (see Chapter Eight, Solving the Pandemic Problem), you know that we can't (or ought not to) remain blissfully unaware of what that means.

So, we might need to become more comfortable asking our doctors and healthcare providers questions when they lapse into jargon we aren't familiar with and be patient with our healthcare providers when we are a bit more ahead of the technological curve than they are. Or use social media as a tool to learn about these topics. Many doctors and scientists use social media to share when they publish a new journal article, often describing it in plain English for the rest of us and providing you with a platform to ask them questions. In sum, it means becoming an active participant in our healthcare and wellness.

And when it comes to the ethical questions that AI brings us, it might mean taking a minute to really think about whether some of these are actually problems for you. After all, we aren't all car mechanics, and tax accountants still do a brisk business in early spring despite the many do-it-yourself tax software programs available. Can you feel comfortable with knowing that AI is making our doctors even better than before without understanding exactly how these programs work?

Are You Ready for the Future?

In this constantly changing field, what can you do now to protect yourself from the potential harms of AI in medicine and wellness?

1. Ask questions! While you probably won't ask the doctor at your next checkup if he's using AI in your care (that might be a little weird), you can pay attention to the healthcare news to learn about new advances in technology. Hospitals often publish patient-oriented magazines, newspapers, or web pages with information about new equipment, programs, or research being done. Stripped of technical jargon, these are a great resource for

learning how your healthcare providers are meeting the challenges I've described throughout this book.

What's more, many doctors and scientists have active social media accounts they use to specifically educate laypersons about new advances. Take advantage of the opportunity to ask them questions.

2. Think about where you stand on topics like gene editing. It's already being used to successfully treat some disorders. If offered the opportunity, would you take it?

3. Make your home network harder to hack. Everything from your Nest Thermostat to the Ring security system and even your connected scale contains valuable information. With the ever-growing number of connected devices, keeping your devices safe is more important than ever.

CHAPTER TEN:

LIVING YOUR BEST LIFE WITH AI

"If you do not think about your future, you cannot have one."—John Galsworthy, Nobel Prize–winning author

"Most people overestimate what they can do in one year and underestimate what they can do in ten years."—Bill Gates, cofounder of Microsoft and philanthropist

It's time to stop thinking of AI as a futuristic fantasy, far removed from our everyday lives. The technology is being implemented right now in homes, hospitals, doctor's offices, pharmacies, and point-of-care clinics across the country. Our gyms and fitness equipment are optimized using AI to help us reach our bucket list goals: running a marathon, hiking the Pacific Coast Trail à la Cheryl Strayed, or bench-pressing our body weight. Want to lose twenty pounds, lower your blood pressure, or finally master yoga? AI can help you with that. Throughout this book, you've learned some of the many ways AI is already impacting our healthcare system and wellness industry, and how it will continue to change the medical landscape for years to come.

But what does it all mean for you, the reader? What do you need to know to take advantage of all AI has to offer in order to improve your health and medical outcomes? Which AI-enabled devices, tests, and treatments should you seek out and how do you find them? Should you look for doctors and healthcare providers who embrace AI, and if so, how do you know which ones do? How do you know when to trust a technology and what is too beta to try? How do you protect your privacy as a patient? And what do you need to know now to prepare yourself for how AI will change healthcare in the future?

This chapter will outline ways you can leverage everything you've learned in the previous nine chapters to navigate the good, bad, and ugly of AI to stay healthy and happy.

My goal is to make the suggestions in this chapter accessible, universal, and applicable to all readers regardless of how healthy you are, what access you have to healthcare providers, what insurance coverage you have, and/or how much money or time you're willing to spend on medical care or fitness programs.

Where We've Been and Where We're Headed

In the past several decades, we have seen multiple vehicles land on Mars, seen photographs of Pluto, and discovered thousands of exoplanets. Scientists put a new branch on our ancestral family tree with the discovery of *Homo naledi* and identified the ruins of Mayan buildings with airborne lasers. But scientific research has also hit much closer to home: we've developed not just one vaccine for a global pandemic, but multiple—in a matter of months. State-of-the-art hospitals manage patients and their heating and air conditioning systems from command centers that are light years different from the wards of the past. And we're using our smartphones, smartwatches, fitness, and health trackers to help us get or stay in shape, relax, and sleep better.

Behind these advances is technology that improves by the day. Artificial intelligence, once the stuff of sci-fi movies and fantasy, is already here. Machine learning algorithms predict who will develop invasive breast cancer more than a year before a radiologist will be able to see it on a mammogram. EHR systems alert doctors to patients who are at risk of sepsis and who have undiagnosed diabetes. Virtual reality workouts let us feel like we're in a yoga class on a beach in Bali, rock climbing El Capitan, or in the boxing ring with Ali—all from our house in the middle of a blizzard. We can use an AI chatbot to provide mental health counseling or guide us in a personalized meditation.

If you were to look at healthcare from thirty thousand feet, you might think that things are running pretty much as they did decades ago. People check in with their doctors once a year or so for an annual exam; when they get really sick, they head to the hospital. Doctors prescribe medicine to help us get better and to treat chronic diseases. From this viewpoint, things don't look very different. But if you were to take a deep dive into any one of those things, you'd get a very different opinion.

Our doctors' appointments are just as likely (or even more so) to take place using our phones, tablets, or computers as they are to happen in an office. We can be sitting on the beach on vacation and grab a quick appointment to find out if our earache is an infection or simply the result of a plane ride. Our healthcare providers don't need to be tied to their offices either.

Labs can be ordered online, and we can head to the nearest pharmacy or grocery store for a blood draw on our schedule. If we get really sick outside of normal office hours or injure ourselves, we can head to the nearest urgent care location or clinic inside a pharmacy or grocery store, where we can be treated more quickly than at the emergency room. Video consults by specialists mean we don't have to sacrifice quality care for convenience.

When we need a prescription, it might just as easily involve an app as a pill bottle. Our medicine is becoming ever more personalized: drugs based on our unique genomic information, not simply what condition we have. Pharmaceutical companies are cutting years off of the drug development process, getting lifesaving and quality-of-life–improving medications to us quicker than ever before.

Smartphones, smartwatches, computers, big data … close-up, our healthcare looks nothing like the system of yesterday. There is truly not one aspect of our lives that isn't impacted by AI. Everything from the food we eat, to the clothes we wear, to the things we do for work and for fun—AI is behind it and here to stay.

Navigating Today's World from an AI Perspective

You don't need to have a medical degree or be a computer science genius to take control of your health and wellness in ways you probably never thought of or thought could really work. AI is leveling the playing field by bringing the power of technology to the masses.

In Chapter Three, I showed you a dozen examples that can be used to improve your health using your smartphone. You now know that your smartphone is just the tip of the iceberg when it comes to you and AI.

After reading the previous chapters, if you still feel that this "Future" of AI in healthcare is still some time off, or that the things I describe aren't going to have a real impact for a few years, let me show you otherwise.

Telemedicine became the standard way for most people to see their doctors during the COVID-19 pandemic. It's probably not going away anytime soon—at least for some healthcare providers. Genetic counselors or mental health professionals have been delivering care via telephone and more recently by video calls for several years already. And that's good for everyone. Instead of being resigned to traveling to an office when you're already feeling under the weather or trying to squeeze a routine checkup or therapy appointment into your busy day, telemedicine is making it easier for patients to receive the care they need when it's more convenient for them.

For people who work atypical hours, including healthcare professionals and first responders on night shifts, or simply anyone who is unable to make health appointments during normal business hours, telemedicine is an opportunity to fit in healthcare on their schedule. Providers who live in different time zones (or those who prefer to work different hours) can deliver care that doesn't require an in-person exam or lab work.

Despite overall positive experiences from patients and providers with telemedicine, whether it will remain an option for everyone is up for debate. Weighing in on the debate by contacting your legislators could have real consequences in the immediate future.

If I had written on the first page of this book that scientists have created a *Star Trek* tricorder, that we can cure disease by rewriting our DNA, and that we can create a vaccine against a newly discovered virus in a tenth of the time it normally takes, you might have been skeptical. But those are things that not only are possible—you've seen that they're already here.

One of the most important takeaways I hope you get from this book is that the technology I've described, the companies and apps I highlighted, are really just the tip of the iceberg. Do you want to learn more about gene editing? Or pharmacogenomic tests? Or which apps to download today to get into shape before summer? Even if I could create a comprehensive list of all of the resources where you could go to get that information, chances are that within a few weeks, it would be outdated. (The appendix has a variety of sources, arranged by chapter, including links to peer-reviewed scientific papers, if you want to start there.) So, while I've provided some examples, I can't recommend enough that you continue learning more about the topics that interest you the most. Starting with the examples I provided is a good first step. If you're anything like me, once you start down the rabbit hole of learning, it's hard to get out. ☺

The Future You: The Future is Now

Instead of a checklist, this book is meant as more of a guidebook. Just like you might check out Rick Steves's books before heading to Paris or Madrid, *The Future You* can be your guidebook to how AI and big data are transforming healthcare. It's a little bit of the roadmap of how we move away from the focus of healthcare as "care for the sick" to wellness care—how we stay healthy and well in the first place to avoid disease. That's a radical transformation—and while there's a lot of interest in getting to the end result, it's hard work, and there are many barriers in the way. I think AI is going to help us get there sooner and remove some of those roadblocks.

Getting to the Future You doesn't look the same for everyone. What works for me (controlling the sleep apnea my Apple Watch picked up on, staying on the keto diet, getting better, more restful sleep) isn't even the same as what will work for my wife, who might want to eat a bagel once in a while and is better at meditation than I am. But here are few of my thoughts to help you think about what *The Future You* means for you.

1. Did you read Chapter Six and ask yourself if you could sequence your entire genome and have it interpreted by an expert for $100 whether would you jump on the opportunity? Costs of genetic testing and sequencing have dropped dramatically over the past decade, and genetic testing is now standard of care for some conditions and for patients diagnosed with cancer. I've described how testing can inform doctors about potential adverse effects of some drugs due to specific genetic differences that can make you a faster, or slower, metabolizer of certain medications. Genetic tests are used to determine which chemotherapy a cancer patient has the best chance of benefiting from. Liquid biopsies are helping to make repeat, painful tissue biopsies a thing of the past.

2. Did reading Chapter Four make you wonder about what devices you'd want to have now or in the future? Things like connected scales or blood pressure monitors? Not only can you use those devices now to see trends over time, but the information could be valuable if you get sick. Remember Anthony Purser? He's the Houston man I wrote about in the Introduction who used the ECG data from his Apple Watch to prove he

was having atrial fibrillation—information that was then used to get him the right treatment, getting him back to his normal routines.

3. Feel overwhelmed by the sheer number of things that were in Chapter Three? Picking a platform that integrates all of your health and fitness data into a single, easy-to-access app or website might be the choice for you. Apple, Google, Samsung, and Fitbit (now part of Google) are all popular options. And if you're in the mood for something new or want a challenge, fitness platforms like Strava or MapMyFitness can give you an online community and goals to improve your health, workout routine, or nutrition.

4. Worried about COVID-19 or the next pandemic lurking around the corner? I hope that Chapter Eight helped you feel a little more confident that scientists will be even better prepared. AI is being used around the world by public health officials to monitor potential outbreaks. We've just seen the global scientific community come together to identify the pathogen and use AI to develop multiple vaccines in record time. While there's always concern for a previously unknown virus to jump from its animal reservoir into humans, COVID-19 laid the groundwork for how to handle it.

5. And if you were worried about how scientists could develop a vaccine for COVID-19 when most medications take more than a decade to reach consumers, Chapter Seven should have allayed at least some of your fears. AI is helping pharmaceutical companies blast through preclinical research faster than ever before. Only AI could help scientists read through all of the

scientific literature and comb through the millions
of potential small molecules and drug targets so
quickly. And as I described, it's also helping to
make clinical trials more accessible, through
remote monitoring of patients and through "digital
twins" who serve as the placebo. The rapidity at
which the vaccines were developed is incredible—
and it would be inappropriate to think that all new
drugs could enjoy the same timetable. But we
should start to see the decade-long timeframe
shrink considerably and (hopefully) alongside that,
the costs.

6. Wonder how your hospital can stack up against
   such AI-powered centers as the Humber River
   Hospital in Ontario (see Chapter Four)? Even
   though Boston has some of the world's best
   hospitals, it's not hard to be a little envious of
   patients who can experience top-quality care in
   such an automated, efficient, and futuristic
   environment. The good news is that top quality
   healthcare doesn't have to wait. Even community
   hospitals in rural settings across the US can benefit
   from AI—and it may help cut costs.

7. If you know someone with a rare disease, someone
   with cancer, or really, anyone with a health
   condition, it might have been hard to read Chapter
   Five and not think of how great it would be to use
   gene editing to fix it. AI is doing remarkable things
   for so many conditions, it's difficult to keep up
   with each new press release. Take blindness, for
   example. Scientists using CRISPR to treat a
   hereditary form of blindness found that treating
   one eye actually improved sight in the patient's
   second (untreated) eye! And we're getting better at
   diagnosing and predicting the clinical course of
   patients with diabetic retinopathy, glaucoma, and

age-related macular degeneration, diseases that are responsible for blindness in millions of adults. Other diseases and health conditions aren't far behind.

8. While Chapter One was designed to ease you into thinking about AI technology by showing you how it's being used in nonhealthcare ways, I hope it spurs your thinking about situations I didn't even mention. The XPRIZE Foundation, backers of the tricorder challenge (Chapter Three), held a global learning challenge to find new technologies to help children around the world learn, at their own pace, the basics of reading, writing, and arithmetic (https://www.xprize.org/prizes/global-learning). Spoiler alert: AI plays a big role in the solutions. And it's not just healthcare, agriculture, manufacturing, education … AI is literally—yes, I do mean *literally*—impacting every industry today. It might not be at the same level across the board, but nothing we do, eat, drink, watch, etc. isn't impacted, mostly in a positive way, by this technology.

So, what will the Future You look like? Will we have smartphones that contain all of the data from the various other tech devices we own, or will we, human beings, be augmented with technology and wearables that take the place of the ubiquitous device? Will we see the average human lifespan grow from eighty-something to more than one hundred as we preemptively address diseases like cancer through gene editing and predictive analytics? Will we forego annual visits to the doctor and instead use smart clothing and our connected devices to continually track our health, nutrition, and mental well-being? Will the office visits we have be entirely remote and taken from our comfy couch in front of our smart TV and our relevant health data from our devices already uploaded to our electronic health record, ready for an AI algorithm to find the trends and recommend what we should do to improve? I don't have a crystal ball, but these scenarios sound not that far off, considering what we are already capable of.

The real question is what will you do? It's time to take charge of your future well-being.

☺You're in control on the path to *The Future You*.

REFERENCES

The following references are meant to provide you with some options in case you would like to learn more about any of the topics described in this book. They are arranged by chapter and most include website links. When direct links for scientific papers can't be found or the website charges a subscription fee, I recommend using Pubmed (http://pubmed.ncbi.nlm.nih.gov). Many of the papers are freely available through Pubmed, and you'll be able to find other scientific papers on the same topics, should you want to take a deeper dive.

Introduction

Alba, D. (2016). Zuckerberg and Chan Promise $3 Billion to Cure Every Disease. *Wired*. Retrieved from https://www.wired.com/2016/09/zuckerberg-chan-promise-3-billion-curing-disease/

Apple. (2015). Apple Introduces ResearchKit, Giving Medical Researchers the Tools to Revolutionize Medical Studies [Press release]. Retrieved from https://www.apple.com/newsroom/2015/03/09Apple-Introduces-ResearchKit-Giving-Medical-Researchers-the-Tools-to-Revolutionize-Medical-Studies/

Boitnott, J. (2018). Facebook Is Quietly Showcasing the Future of Healthcare—and You Should Pay Attention. *Inc*. Retrieved from https://www.inc.com/john-boitnott/how-facebook-us-government-are-using-artificial-intelligence-to-stop-suicide-drug-addiction.html

Centers for Medicare and Medicaid Services (CMS). (2021, December 16, 2020). National Health Expenditure Data. Retrieved from https://www.cms.gov/Research-Statistics-Data-and-Systems/Statistics-Trends-and-

Reports/NationalHealthExpendData/NationalHealthAcc
ountsHistorical

Dolan, B. (2014). In-Depth: What Apple's Health app
tracks and what it forgot to include. *Mobi Health News*.
Retrieved from
http://www.mobihealthnews.com/34113/in-depth-what-
apples-health-app-tracks-and-what-it-forgot-to-include

Fowler, G. A., & Kelly, H. (2020, December 10, 2020).
Amazon's new health band is the most invasive tech
we've ever tested. *The Washington Post*. Retrieved from
https://www.washingtonpost.com/technology/2020/12
/10/amazon-halo-band-review/

Freedman, D. H. (2019, December 3, 2019). Do You
Trust Jeff Bezos With Your Life? Tech Giants Like
Amazon Are Getting into the Healthcare Business.
Newsweek. Retrieved from
https://www.newsweek.com/amazon-healthcare-jeff-
bezos-telemedicine-1475154

Fussell, S. (2020). The Sneaky Genius of Facebook's New
Preventive Health Tool. *The Atlantic*. Retrieved from
https://www.theatlantic.com/technology/archive/2020/
01/facebook-launches-new-preventative-health-
tool/604567/

Garcia, J. (February 15, 2021). Normal tests couldn't
prove Houston man's irregular heartbeat. But his Apple
Watch could. *Houston Chronicle*. Retrieved from
https://www.houstonchronicle.com/lifestyle/renew-
houston/health/article/Normal-tests-couldn-t-prove-
Houston-man-s-15946059.php

Geer, Michael. (February 15, 2021). What's more
important? Lifespan or Health Span? Retrieved from

https://glorikian.com/whats-more-important-lifespan-or-health-span-michael-geer/

Gurdus, L. (2019). Tim Cook: Apple's greatest contribution will be 'about health'. *CNBC*. Retrieved from https://www.cnbc.com/2019/01/08/tim-cook-teases-new-apple-services-tied-to-health-care.html

Hackett, M. (2020). Oura Ring detects the onset of fever, a common COVID-19 symptom. *Mobi Health News*. Retrieved from https://www.mobihealthnews.com/news/oura-ring-detects-onset-fever-common-covid-19-symptom

Hirten, R. P., Danieletto, M., Tomalin, L., Choi, K. H., Zweig, M., Golden, E., Sparshdeep, K., et al. (2021). Use of Physiological Data From a Wearable Device to Identify SARS-CoV-2 Infection and Symptoms and Predict COVID-19 Diagnosis: Observational Study. *Journal of Medical Internet Research*, 23(2), e26107. doi:10.2196/26107. https://www.jmir.org/2021/2/e26107/

Kent, J. (2018). Facebook, NYU Will Use Artificial Intelligence for Faster MRIs. *Health IT Analytics*. Retrieved from https://healthitanalytics.com/news/facebook-nyu-will-use-artificial-intelligence-for-faster-mris

La Monica, P. R. (2019). Amazon is now the most valuable company on the planet. *CNN*. Retrieved from https://www.cnn.com/2019/01/08/investing/amazon-most-valuable-company-microsoft-google-apple/index.html

Laguarta, J., Hueto, F., Subirana, B. (2020). COVID-19 Artificial Intelligence Diagnosis Using Only Cough Recordings. *IEEE Open Journal of Engineering in Medicine*

and Biology, 1, 275-281.
doi:10.1109/OJEMB.2020.3026928.
https://ieeexplore.ieee.org/document/9208795

Lovett, L. (2018). Study: Apple Watches paired with
Cardiogram can detect a-fib. *Mobi Health News*. Retrieved
from http://www.mobihealthnews.com/content/study-
apple-watches-paired-cardiogram-can-detect-fib

Mayo Clinic Staff. (2021). Atrial Fibrillation. *Mayo Clinic*.
Retrieved from https://www.mayoclinic.org/diseases-
conditions/atrial-fibrillation/symptoms-causes/syc-
20350624

(March 4, 2020). AI, Azure and the future of healthcare
with Dr. Peter Lee. *Microsoft Research*. Retrieved from
https://www.microsoft.com/en-us/research/blog/ai-
azure-and-the-future-of-healthcare-with-dr-peter-lee/

Miliard, M. (2020). Microsoft launches major $40M AI
for Health initiative. *Healthcare IT News*. Retrieved from
https://www.healthcareitnews.com/news/microsoft-
launches-major-40m-ai-health-initiative

Orlandic, L., Teijeiro, T., Atienza, D. (2020). The
COUGHVID crowdsourcing data set: A corpus for the
study of large-scale cough analysis algorithms. *Cornell
University/arXvi.org*. Retrieved from
https://arxiv.org/abs/2009.11644

Reuters. (2020). WEF 2020: Alphabet CEO Pichai eyes
major opportunity in healthcare, says will protect privacy.
Business Today. Retrieved from
https://www.businesstoday.in/wef-2020/news/wef-
2020-alphabet-ceo-pichai-eyes-major-opportunity-in-
healthcare-says-will-protect-privacy/story/394441.html

Smarr, B. L., Aschbacher, K., Fisher, S. M., Chowdhary, A., Dilchert, S., Puldon, K., Rao, A., Hecht, F., Mason, A. E. (2020). Feasibility of continuous fever monitoring using wearable devices. *Scientific Reports*, 10(1), 21640. doi:10.1038/s41598-020-78355-6. https://pubmed.ncbi.nlm.nih.gov/33318528/

Statt, N. (2021). Facebook is secretly building a smartwatch and planning to sell it next year. *The Verge*. Retrieved from https://www.theverge.com/2021/2/12/22280798/facebook-smartwatch-messaging-health-fitness-release-date

Thoreau, H. D. (1908). *Walden; or, Life in the Woods*. London: J. M. Dent. https://www.worldcat.org/title/walden-or-life-in-the-woods/oclc/2514508

Chapter One

AI City Challenge. (2021). *AI City Challenge*. Retrieved from https://www.aicitychallenge.org

Ambalina, L. (2019). Top 10 Vehicle and Cars Datasets for Machine Learning. *Lionbridge AI*. Retrieved from https://lionbridge.ai/datasets/250000-cars-top-10-free-vehicle-image-and-video-datasets-for-machine-learning/

Elezaj, R. (2019). How AI Is Paving the Way for Autonomous Cars. *MachineDesign*. Retrieved from https://www.machinedesign.com/mechanical-motion-systems/article/21838234/how-ai-is-paving-the-way-for-autonomous-cars

Feng, Q., Ablavsky, V., Sclaroff, S. (2021). CityFlow-NL: Tracking and Retrieval of Vehicles at City Scaleby Natural

Language Descriptions. *Cornell University/arXvi.* arXiv preprint arXiv:2101.04741. https://arxiv.org/abs/2101.04741

(February 1, 2021). IntelinAir's AI-Driven Image Analysis is Saving Crops. Retrieved from https://glorikian.com/intelinairs-ai-driven-image-analysis-is-saving-crops-down-on-the-farm-today-but-tomorrow/

Hammond, K. (2017). The Periodic Table of AI. *Data Science Central.* Retrieved from https://www.datasciencecentral.com/profiles/blogs/the-periodic-table-of-ai

Reinhart, R. (2018). Most Americans Already Using Artificial Intelligence Products. *Gallup.* Retrieved from https://news.gallup.com/poll/228497/americans-already-using-artificial-intelligence-products.aspx

Rogers, A. (2018). How Grubhub Analyzed 4,000 Dishes to Predict Your Next Order. *Wired.* Retrieved from https://www.wired.com/story/how-grubhub-analyzed-4000-dishes-to-predict-your-next-order/

Schwab, K. (2017). *The Fourth Industrial Revolution.* New York: Crown Publishing Group.

Tang, Z., Naphade, M., Liu, M-Y., Yang, X., Birchfield, S., Wang, S., Kumar, R., Anastasiu, D., Hwang, J-N. (March 21/April 5, 2019). Cityflow: A city-scale benchmark for multi-target multi-camera vehicle tracking and re-identification. Paper presented at the Proceedings of the IEEE/CVF Conference on Computer Vision and Pattern Recognition. *Cornell University/arXvi.* https://arxiv.org/abs/1903.09254

Walch, K. (2019). How AI is Transforming Agriculture. *Forbes*. Retrieved from https://www.forbes.com/sites/cognitiveworld/2019/07/05/how-ai-is-transforming-agriculture/?sh=1cd681a44ad1

XPRIZE Foundation. (2021). XPRIZE AI Prize Teams. Retrieved from https://www.xprize.org/prizes/artificial-intelligence/teams

Chapter Two

Albrecht, C. (2020). Heali Launches its AI-Based Nutrition and Meal Planning App. *The Spoon*. Retrieved from https://thespoon.tech/heali-launches-its-ai-based-nutrition-and-meal-planning-app/

American Academy of Sleep Medicine. (2020). Insomnia. Retrieved from https://aasm.org/resources/factsheets/insomnia.pdf

Barratt, E. L., Davis, N. J. (2015). Autonomous Sensory Meridian Response (ASMR): a flow-like mental state. *PeerJ*, 3, e851. doi:10.7717/peerj.85. https://peerj.com/articles/851/

Barrett, B., Harden, C. M., Brown, R. L., Coe, C. L., Irwin, M. R. (2020). Mindfulness meditation and exercise both improve sleep quality: Secondary analysis of a randomized controlled trial of community dwelling adults. *Sleep Health*, 6(6), 804-813. doi:10.1016/j.sleh.2020.04.003. https://www.sleephealthjournal.org/article/S2352-7218(20)30115-7/abstract

Centers for Disease Control and Prevention. (2020, May 2, 2017). Sleep and Sleep Disorders. Retrieved from https://www.cdc.gov/sleep/data_statistics.html

Costa, C. (2020). The Peloton threat: Gyms have a plan to get Americans working out again. *CNBC*. Retrieved from https://www.cnbc.com/2020/09/12/peloton-how-gyms-plan-to-get-americans-working-out-again.html

Eight Sleep. (2020). Eight Sleep Technology. Retrieved from https://www.eightsleep.com/technology/

El Morr, C., Ritvo, P., Ahmad, F., Moineddin, R. (2020). Effectiveness of an 8-Week Web-Based Mindfulness Virtual Community Intervention for University Students on Symptoms of Stress, Anxiety, and Depression: Randomized Controlled Trial. *Journal of Medical Internet Research*, 7(7), e18595. doi:10.2196/18595. https://mental.jmir.org/2020/7/e18595/

Grand View Research. (2019). Weight Loss Services Market Size, Share & Trends Report By Payment (Out of Pocket, Private Insurance), By Equipment (Fitness, Surgical), By Services (Consulting, Fitness Center), And Segment Forecasts, 2019-2025. *Grand View Research*. Retrieved from https://www.grandviewresearch.com/industry-analysis/weight-loss-services-market

Hsu, J. (2018). The Strava Heat Map and the End of Secrets. *Wired*. Retrieved from https://www.wired.com/story/strava-heat-map-military-bases-fitness-trackers-privacy/

Hurford, M. (2020). MyFitnessPal's New Meal Scan Features Makes Logging a Snap. *MyFitnessPal*. Retrieved from https://blog.myfitnesspal.com/myfitnesspals-new-meal-scan-feature-makes-logging-a-snap/

Kuzma, C. (2020). Secrets to Perfecting Your On-the-Run Art. *Runner's World*. Retrieved from https://www.runnersworld.com/runners-stories/a32433537/strava-art/

Lee, M., Song, C. B., Shin, G. H., Lee, S. W. (2019). Possible Effect of Binaural Beat Combined With Autonomous Sensory Meridian Response for Inducing Sleep. *Frontiers in Human Neuroscience*, 13, 425. doi:10.3389/fnhum.2019.00425. https://www.frontiersin.org/articles/10.3389/fnhum.2019.00425/full#:~:text=10.3389%2Ffnhum.2019.00425-,Possible%20Effect%20of%20Binaural%20Beat%20Combined%20With,Meridian%20Response%20for%20Inducing%20Sleep&text=Sleep%20is%20important%20to%20maintain,diso

Passman, J. (2016). The World's Most Relaxing Song. *Forbes*. Retrieved from https://www.forbes.com/sites/jordanpassman/2016/11/23/the-worlds-most-relaxing-song/?sh=6ce2c4812053

Perez, S., & Lunden, I. (2018). Meditation app Headspace bets on voice and AI with Alpine.AI acquisition. *Tech Crunch*. Retrieved from https://techcrunch.com/2018/09/04/meditation-app-headspace-bets-on-voice-and-a-i-with-alpine-ai-acquisition/

Rest Performance. (2020). ReST Sleep Technology. Retrieved from https://restperformance.com/sleep-tech/

Rowland, M. P. (2018). Beyoncé is Using Artificial Intelligence to Help You Eat Vegan. *Forbes*. Retrieved from https://www.forbes.com/sites/michaelpellmanrowland/2018/04/24/beyonce-artificial-intelligence-vegan/?sh=40483ecb7160

Settembre, J. (2018). This is the insane amount millenials are spending on fitness. *MarketWatch*. Retrieved from https://www.marketwatch.com/story/this-is-the-insane-amount-millennials-are-spending-on-fitness-2018-01-21

Sleep Number. (2021). Sleep Number i8 bed. Retrieved from https://www.sleepnumber.com/products/i8

Strava. (2021). Strava Heat Map. Retrieved from https://www.strava.com/heatmap#13.86/-73.57981/41.30926/hot/all

Terlep, S. (2020, June 30, 2020). Lululemon Buys Mirror, an At-Home Fitness Start-up, for $500 Million. *The Wall Street Journal*. Retrieved from https://www.wsj.com/articles/lululemon-to-buy-at-home-fitness-company-mirror-for-500-million-11593465981

Tilghman, A. (2016). The Pentagon has banned Pokemon Go from official military phones. *Military Times*. Retrieved from https://www.militarytimes.com/news/your-military/2016/08/12/the-pentagon-has-banned-pokemon-go-from-official-military-phones/

VR Electronics Ltd. (2021). Teslasuit. Retrieved from https://teslasuit.io

Chapter Three

Apple. (2006). Nike and Apple Team Up to Launch Nike+iPod [Press release]. Retrieved from https://www.apple.com/newsroom/2006/05/23Nike-and-Apple-Team-Up-to-Launch-Nike-iPod/

Apple. (2015). Apple Announces ResearchKit Available Today to Medical Researchers [Press release]. Retrieved from https://www.apple.com/newsroom/2015/04/14Apple-Announces-ResearchKit-Available-Today-to-Medical-Researchers/

Apple. (2016). Apple Advances Health Apps with CareKit [Press release]. Retrieved from https://www.apple.com/newsroom/2016/03/21Apple-Advances-Health-Apps-with-CareKit/

Apple. (2017). Apple Heart Study launches to identify irregular heart rhythms. Retrieved from https://www.apple.com/newsroom/2017/11/apple-heart-study-launches-to-identify-irregular-heart-rhythms/

Belfiore, M. (June 22, 2015). Tricorder XPRIZE Competition Heats Up. *Scientific American*. Retrieved from https://www.scientificamerican.com/article/tricorder-xprize-competition-heats-up/

Brown, P. (2021). The Future of Healthcare May Reside in Your Smart Clothes. Mous4r Electronics. Retrieved from https://www.mouser.com/applications/healthcare-may-reside-in-smart-clothing/

Byambasuren, O., Beller, E., Glasziou, P. (2019). Current Knowledge and Adoption of Mobile Health Apps Among Australian General Practitioners: Survey Study. *Journal of Medical Internet Research (JMIR Mhealth Uhealth)*, 7(6), e13199. doi:10.2196/13199. https://pubmed.ncbi.nlm.nih.gov/31199343/

Carroll, L., Reuters Health. (2018). Smartphone app could screen for anemia. Retrieved from https://www.reuters.com/article/us-health-anemia-smartphones/smartphone-app-could-screen-for-anemia-idUSKBN1O42R8

Centers for Disease Control and Prevention. (March 9, 2020). Opioid Overdose. Retrieved from https://www.cdc.gov/drugoverdose/epidemic/index.html

Centers for Disease Control and Prevention. (2021, July 26, 2018). Healthy Contact Lens Wear and Care. Retrieved from https://www.cdc.gov/contactlenses/fast-facts.html

Chan, P. H., Wong, C. K., Poh, Y. C., Pun, L., Leung, W. W., Wong, Y., Wong, M. M., Poh, M., Chu, D. W., Siu, C. (2016). Diagnostic Performance of a Smartphone-Based Photoplethysmographic Application for Atrial Fibrillation Screening in a Primary Care Setting. *Journal of the American Heart Association*, 5(7). doi:10.1161/jaha.116.003428. https://www.ahajournals.org/doi/10.1161/JAHA.116.003428

Cloud DX. (2020). Cloud DX Announces Connected Health Kit and Rapid Deployment Program for COVID-19 Remote Patient Monitoring [Press release]. *Cision PR Newswire*. Retrieved from https://www.prnewswire.com/news-releases/cloud-dx-announces-connected-health-kit-and-rapid-deployment-program-for-covid-19-remote-patient-monitoring-301135613.html

Cooling, G. (2020). Apple Introduces Hearing Aid Like Features For Their Airpods Pro with New IOS Update. Retrieved from https://www.hearingaidknow.com/hearing-aid-functionality-introduced-to-apple-airpods-pro

Crum, P. (2019). Hearables Will Monitor Your Brain and Body to Augment Your Life. *IEEE Spectrum*. Retrieved from https://spectrum.ieee.org/consumer-electronics/audiovideo/hearables-will-monitor-your-brain-and-body-to-augment-your-life

Daré Bioscience. (2021). DARE-LARC1 — User-controlled, long-acting reversible contraception. Retrieved from https://darebioscience.com/microchips-biotech/

Garcia, L. M., Birckhead, B. J., Krishnamurthy, P., Sackman, J., Mackey, I. G., Louis, R. G., Salmasi, V., Maddox, T., Darnall, B. D. (2021). An 8-Week Self-Administered At-Home Behavioral Skills-Based Virtual Reality Program for Chronic Low Back Pain: Double-Blind, Randomized, Placebo-Controlled Trial Conducted During COVID-19. *Journal of Medical Internet Research*, 23(2), e26292. doi:10.2196/26292. https://www.jmir.org/2021/2/e26292/

Joyce, M., Leclerc, O., Westhues, K., Xue, H. (2018). Digital therapeutics: Preparing for takeoff. Retrieved from https://www.mckinsey.com/industries/pharmaceuticals-and-medical-products/our-insights/digital-therapeutics-preparing-for-takeoff

Khalid, A. (2020). Pulse oximeters are selling out because of the pandemic. Most people don't need them. *Quartz*. Retrieved from https://qz.com/1832464/pulse-oximeters-for-coronavirus-unnecessary-but-selling-strong/

Kong, Y. L., Zou, X., McCandler, C. A., Kirtane, A. R., Ning, S., Zhou, J., Abid, A., Jafarie, M., Rogner, J., Traverso, G. (2019). 3D-Printed Gastric Resident Electronics. Advanced Materials Technologies, 4(3), 1800490. https://doi.org/10.1002/admt.201800490

Ligon, L. (2019). Woman has no doubt Apple Watch saved her life. *Fox 10 News*. Retrieved from https://www.fox10tv.com/news/daily_dot_com/woman-has-no-doubt-apple-watch-saved-her-life/article_9413de32-c5e6-11e9-b8d7-576efea7e2bf.html

Linder, C. (November 22, 2019). If You've Ever Wanted a Smartphone Microscope, Now's Your Chance. *Popular Mechanics*. Retrieved from https://www.popularmechanics.com/technology/gear/a29873640/smartphone-microscope-diple/

Mariakakis, A., Banks, M. A., Phillipi, L., Yu, L., Taylor, J., Patel, S. N. (2017). Biliscreen: smartphone-based scleral jaundice monitoring for liver and pancreatic disorders. Proceedings of the ACM on Interactive, Mobile, Wearable and Ubiquitous Technologies, 1(2), 1-26.

mc10. (2021). Introducing BioStamp nPoint. *MC10*. Retrieved from https://www.mc10inc.com

McQuate, S. (2019). First smartphone app to detect opioid overdose and its precursors. *University of Washington/UW News*. Retrieved from https://www.washington.edu/news/2019/01/09/smartphone-app-detects-opioid-overdose/

McSweeney, K. (2020). The E Tattoo Is the Future of Healthcare Technology. Retrieved from https://now.northropgrumman.com/e-tattoos-are-futuristic-healthcare-wearables

Medtronic. (2021). Pillcam SB3 System. Retrieved from https://www.medtronic.com/covidien/en-us/products/capsule-endoscopy/pillcam-sb-3-system.html

ModernBiz. (2019). Cloud DX, the start-up warping us into a healthier future. Retrieved from https://cloudblogs.microsoft.com/industry-blog/en-ca/uncategorized/2019/05/05/cloud-dx-the-startup-warping-us-into-a-healthier-future/

Morin, C. M. (2020). Profile of Somryst Prescription Digital Therapeutic for Chronic Insomnia: Overview of Safety and Efficacy. *Expert Review of Medical Devices*, 17(12), 1239-1248. doi:10.1080/17434440.2020.1852929. https://www.tandfonline.com/doi/full/10.1080/174344 40.2020.1852929

Murph, D. (2011). Withings fittingly debuts iPhone-connected blood pressure monitor at CES. *Engadget*. Retrieved from https://www.engadget.com/2011-01-04-withings-fittingly-debuts-iphone-connected-blood-pressure-monito.html

Neuralink. (2021). Breakthrough Technology for the Brain. Retrieved from https://neuralink.com

Novartis. (2018). Novartis and Pear Therapeutics to develop digital therapeutics for patients with schizophrenia and multiple sclerosis [Press release]. Retrieved from https://www.novartis.com/news/media-releases/novartis-and-pear-therapeutics-develop-digital-therapeutics-patients-schizophrenia-and-multiple-sclerosis

O'Hara, A. (2019). Apple Watch credited with saving life of Seattle man with AFib. Retrieved from https://appleinsider.com/articles/19/02/21/apple-watch-credited-with-saving-life-of-seattle-man-with-afib

Park, J., Kim, J., Kim, S-Y., Cheong, W. H., Jang, J., Park, Y-G., Na, K., et al. (2018). Soft, smart contact lenses with integrations of wireless circuits, glucose sensors, and displays. *Science Advances*, 4(1), eaap9841.

doi:10.1126/sciadv.aap9841.
https://advances.sciencemag.org/content/4/1/eaap9841

Parshley, L. (2020). Our phones can now detect health problems from Parkinson's to depression. Is that a good thing? *Vox*. Retrieved from https://www.vox.com/the-highlight/2020/2/5/21056921/phones-health-apps-data-digital-phenotyping

Perez, M. V., Mahaffey, K. W., Hedlin, H., Rumsfeld, J. S., Garcia, A., Ferris, T., Balasubramian, et al. (2019). Large-Scale Assessment of a Smartwatch to Identify Atrial Fibrillation. *New England Journal of Medicine,* 381(20), 1909-1917. doi:10.1056/NEJMoa1901183. https://www.nejm.org/doi/full/10.1056/NEJMoa1901183

Pew Research Center. (2019). Mobile Fact Sheet. Retrieved from http://www.pewInternet.org/fact-sheet/mobile/

Picheta, R. (2020). Apps that claim to test moles are missing skin cancers, doctors warn. *CNN*. Retrieved from https://www.cnn.com/2020/02/10/health/skin-cancer-melanoma-apps-study-wellness-scli-intl/index.html

Pierce, D. (2017). The iPhone's Turning 10. What will it look like at 20? *Wired*. Retrieved from https://www.wired.com/story/imagining-the-iphone-in-2027/

Pogue, D. (December 19, 2017). How Good Is *Star Trek*'s Record at Predicting the Future of Tech? *Scientific American*. Retrieved from https://www.scientificamerican.com/article/how-good-is-star-treks-record-at-predicting-the-future-of-tech/

PreScouter Inc. (2021). The present and future of ingestible sensors—The new taste of science. Retrieved from https://www.prescouter.com/2019/01/ingestible-sensors-innovations/

Rosoff, M. (2014). Your Phone is More Powerful Than the Computer in the Spaceship NASA Launched This Week. *Business Insider.* Retrieved from https://www.businessinsider.com/your-phone-is-more-powerful-than-the-orion-computer-2014-12

Sanyal, S. (2018). Are Hearables The New Wearables Revolutionizing Healthcare? *Forbes.* Retrieved from https://www.forbes.com/sites/shourjyasanyal/2018/11/26/are-hearables-the-new-wearables-revolutionizing-healthcare/#54da4726674b

Senseonics Inc. (2021). Eversense Continuous Glucose Monitoring System. Retrieved from https://www.eversensediabetes.com

Shapiro, A., Bradshaw, B., Landes, S., Kammann, P., Bois De Fer, B., Lee, W-N., Lange, R. (2021). A novel digital approach to describe real world outcomes among patients with constipation. *npj Digital Medicine*, 4(1), 27. doi:10.1038/s41746-021-00391-x. https://www.nature.com/articles/s41746-021-00434-3

Shapiro, A., Marinsek, N., Clay, I., Bradshaw, B., Ramirez, E., Min, J., Trister, A., Wang, Y., Althoff, T., Foschini, L. (2021). Characterizing COVID-19 and Influenza Illnesses in the Real World via Person-Generated Health Data. Patterns, 2(1). *ScienceDirect.* doi:10.1016/j.patter.2020.100188. https://www.sciencedirect.com/science/article/pii/S2666389920302580

Singer, N. (2018, March 18, 2018). Take this app and call me in the morning. *The New York Times*. Retrieved from https://www.nytimes.com/2018/03/18/technology/take-this-app-and-call-me-in-the-morning.html

Statista. (2021). Number of smartphone users worldwide from 2016 to 2021. Retrieved from https://www.statista.com/statistics/330695/number-of-smartphone-users-worldwide/

Stein, R. (October 14, 2004). Implantable Medical ID Approved FDA. *The Washington Post*. Retrieved from https://www.washingtonpost.com/archive/politics/2004/10/14/implantable-medical-id-approved-fda/19ebca25-fb3e-43db-b6b7-7f843ce26daf/

Topol, E. J. (2015). *The Patient Will See You Now: The Future of Medicine is in Your Hands*. New York, NY: Basic Books. https://www.basicbooks.com/titles/eric-topol-md/the-patient-will-see-you-now/9780465040025/

Udrea, A., Mitra, G. D., Costea, D., Noels, E. C., Wakkee, M., Siegel, D. M., de Carvalho, T. M., Nijsten, T. E. C. (2020). Accuracy of a smartphone application for triage of skin lesions based on machine learning algorithms. *Journal of the European Academy of Dermatology and Venereology*, 34(3), 648-655. doi:10.1111/jdv.15935. https://europepmc.org/article/med/31494983

Ugalmugle, S., Swain, R. (2021). mHealth Market Size by Platform ... etc . *Global Market Insights*. Retrieved from https://www.gminsights.com/industry-analysis/mhealth-market

Wagner, A. (2017). Asthma patients breathe easier with new bluetooth inhalers. *PBS*. Retrieved from https://www.pbs.org/newshour/health/asthma-patients-breathe-easier-new-bluetooth-inhalers

Wilson-Anumudu, F., Quan, R., Castro Sweet, C., Cerrada, C., Juusola, J., Turken, M., Bradner Jasik, C. (2021). Early Insights From a Digitally Enhanced Diabetes Self-Management Education and Support Program: Single-Arm Nonrandomized Trial. *Journal of Medical Internet Research Diabetes*, 6(1), e25295. doi:10.2196/25295.
https://diabetes.jmir.org/2021/1/e25295

XPRIZE Foundation. (2021). Empowering Personal Healthcare. Retrieved from
https://www.xprize.org/prizes/tricorder

XPRIZE Foundation. (2021). Qualcomm Tricorder XPrize Cloud DX. Retrieved from
https://www.xprize.org/prizes/tricorder/teams/clouddx

Yarnitsky, D., Dodick, D. W., Grosberg, B. M., Burstein, R., Ironi, A., Harris, D., Lin, T., Silberstein, S. D. (2019). Remote Electrical Neuromodulation (REN) Relieves Acute Migraine: A Randomized, Double-Blind, Placebo-Controlled, Multicenter Trial. Headache: *The Journal of Head and Face Pain*, 59(8), 1240-1252. doi:https://doi.org/10.1111/head.13551.
https://pubmed.ncbi.nlm.nih.gov/31074005/

Chapter Four

American Hospital Association. (2018). Annual Survey IT Supplement Brief #2: Sharing Health Information for Treatment. Retrieved from
https://www.aha.org/system/files/2018-03/sharing-health-information.pdf

American Well. (2016). American Well, CVS Health and Cleveland Clinic Partner to Deliver On-Demand Care to

Healthcare Consumers [Press release]. Retrieved from
https://business.amwell.com/press-release/american-
well-cvs-health-and-cleveland-clinic-partner-to-deliver-
on-demand-care-to-healthcare-consumers/

Bannow, T. (2019). CVS to aggressively expand
healthcare services in stores. *Modern Healthcare*. Retrieved
from https://www.modernhealthcare.com/patient-
care/cvs-aggressively-expand-healthcare-services-stores

Bartlett, J. (2019). Partners, GE say they've developed a
better artificial intelligence. *Boston Business Journal*.
Retrieved from
https://www.bizjournals.com/boston/news/2019/11/26
/partners-ge-say-theyve-developed-a-better.html

Bücking, T. M., Hill, E. R., Robertson, J. L., Maneas, E.,
Plumb, A. A., Nikitichev, D. I. (2017). From medical
imaging data to 3D printed anatomical models. *PLOS
One*, 12(5), e0178540. doi:10.1371/journal.pone.0178540.
https://journals.plos.org/plosone/article?id=10.1371/jou
rnal.pone.0178540

Cantillon, D. J., Loy, M., Burkle, A., Pengel, S.,
Brosovich, D., Hamilton, A., Khot, U., Lindsay, B. D.
(2016). Association Between Off-site Central Monitoring
Using Standardized Cardiac Telemetry and Clinical
Outcomes Among Non–Critically Ill Patients. *The Journal
of the American Medical Association*, 316(5), 519-524.
doi:10.1001/jama.2016.10258.
https://jamanetwork.altmetric.com/details/10213175

Cleveland Clinic. (2019). Combining Nature and
Technology, Luye Medical and Cleveland Clinic Join to
Build a Future Hospital in Shanghai [Press release].
Retrieved from
https://newsroom.clevelandclinic.org/2019/09/20/com
bining-nature-and-technology-luye-medical-and-

cleveland-clinic-join-to-build-a-future-hospital-in-shanghai/

Craven, V. D. (2019). How Technology Saves This Hospital $3.2 Million a Year in Energy Costs. *Buildings*. Retrieved from https://www.buildings.com/news/industry-news/articleid/22162/title/how-technology-saves-hospital

Datta, R., Chon, S. H., Dratsch, T., Timmermann, F., Müller, L., Plum, P. S., Haneder, S., et al. (2020). Are gamers better laparoscopic surgeons? Impact of gaming skills on laparoscopic performance in "Generation Y" students. *PLOS One*, 15(8), e0232341. doi:10.1371/journal.pone.0232341. https://journals.plos.org/plosone/article/comments?id=10.1371/journal.pone.0232341

Dietsche, E. (2017). CVS, Cleveland Clinic expand affiliation as pharmacy-health system collaborations catch on. *MedCity News*. Retrieved from https://medcitynews.com/2017/07/cvs-cleveland-clinic/

Fuentes, L. (2021). The Most Common 3D Printed Prosthetics in 2021. Retrieved from https://all3dp.com/2/the-most-common-3d-printed-prosthetics/

GE (General Electric) (2020). Health Canada Licenses First Artificial Intelligence Algorithms Embedded On-Device to Prioritize Critical Chest X-ray Review [Press release]. Retrieved from https://www.ge.com/news/press-releases/health-canada-licenses-first-artificial-intelligence-algorithms-embedded-device

(2021). Shane Cooke Explains Why Intensive Care Unit Doctors Need a Dashboard. Retrieved from https://glorikian.com/doctors-inintensive-care-units-need-dashboards-explains-shane-cooke/

Gupta, R., Krishnam, S. P., Schaefer, P. W., Lev, M. H., Gilberto Gonzalez, R. (2020). An East Coast Perspective on Artificial Intelligence and Machine Learning: Part 1: Hemorrhagic Stroke Imaging and Triage. *Neuroimaging Clinics of North America Journal*, 30(4), 459-466. doi:10.1016/j.nic.2020.07.005. https://www.neuroimaging.theclinics.com/article/S1052-5149(20)30055-1/abstract

Health and Human Services. Organ Donation Statistics. Retrieved from https://www.organdonor.gov/statistics-stories/statistics.html

Li, D. R., Brennan, J. J., Kreshak, A. A., Castillo, E. M., Vilke, G. M. (2019). Patients Who Leave the Emergency Department Without Being Seen and Their Follow-Up Behavior: A Retrospective Descriptive Analysis. *The Journal of Emergency Medicine*, 57(1), 106-113. doi:10.1016/j.jemermed.2019.03.051. https://www.jem-journal.com/article/S0736-4679(19)30258-6/abstract

Marescaux, J., Leroy, J., Gagner, M., Rubino, F., Mutter, D., Vix, M., Butner, S. E., Smith, M. K. (2001). Transatlantic robot-assisted telesurgery. *Nature*, 413(6854), 379-380. doi:10.1038/35096636. https://www.nature.com/articles/35096636

Parikh, R. (2018). AI can't replace doctors. But it can make them better. *MIT Technology Review*. Retrieved from https://www.technologyreview.com/2018/10/23/139414/ai-cant-replace-doctors-but-it-can-make-them-better/

Rosser, J. C., Jr., Lynch, P. J., Cuddihy, L., Gentile, D. A., Klonsky, J., Merrell, R. (2007). The impact of video games on training surgeons in the 21st century. *The Archives of Surgery/The Journal of the American Medical Association*, 142(2), 181-186; discussion 186. doi:10.1001/archsurg.142.2.181. https://jamanetwork.com/journals/jamasurgery/fullarticl e/399740

Siwicki, B. (2017). Walgreens partners with New York-Presbyterian to offer in-store telemedicine. *Healthcare IT News*. Retrieved from https://www.healthcareitnews.com/news/walgreens-partners-newyork-presbyterian-offer-store-telemedicine

The Medical Futurist. (2020). Where Are 3D-Printed Casts? Retrieved from https://medicalfuturist.com/where-are-3d-printed-casts/

The Medical Futurist. (2021). 5 Reasons Why Artificial Intelligence Won't Replace Physicians. Retrieved from https://medicalfuturist.com/5-reasons-artificial-intelligence-wont-replace-physicians/

Weinick, R. M., Burns, R. M., Mehrotra, A. (2010). Many emergency department visits could be managed at urgent care centers and retail clinics. *Health Affairs* (Millwood), 29(9), 1630-1636. doi:10.1377/hlthaff.2009.0748. https://www.healthaffairs.org/doi/10.1377/hlthaff.2009. 0748

Yasinski, E. (2020). On the Road to 3D Printed Organs. *TheScientist*. Retrieved from https://www.the-scientist.com/news-opinion/on-the-road-to-3-d-printed-organs-67187

Zemmar, A., Lozano, A. M., Nelson, B. J. (2020). The rise of robots in surgical environments during COVID-19.

Nature Machine Intelligence, 2(10), 566-572.
doi:10.1038/s42256-020-00238-2.
https://www.nature.com/articles/s42256-020-00238-2

Chapter Five

Adli, M. (2018). The CRISPR tool kit for genome editing and beyond. *Nature Communications*, 9(1), 1911.
doi:10.1038/s41467-018-04252-2.
https://www.nature.com/articles/s41467-018-04252-2

Alix-Panabières, C., Pantel, K. (2016). Clinical Applications of Circulating Tumor Cells and Circulating Tumor DNA as Liquid Biopsy. *American Association for Cancer Research/Cancer Discovery*, 6(5), 479-491.
doi:10.1158/2159-8290.Cd-15-1483.
https://cancerdiscovery.aacrjournals.org/content/6/5/4
79

Barrangou, R., Doudna, J. A. (2016). Applications of CRISPR technologies in research and beyond. *Nature Biotechnology*, 34(9), 933-941. doi:10.1038/nbt.3659.
https://www.nature.com/articles/nbt.3659

Berg, J. S., Agrawal, P. B., Bailey, D. B., Jr., Beggs, A. H., Brenner, S. E., Brower, A. M., Cakici, J., et al. (2017). Newborn Sequencing in Genomic Medicine and Public Health. *Pediatrics*, 139(2). doi:10.1542/peds.2016-2252.
https://pediatrics.aappublications.org/content/early/201
7/01/15/peds.2016-2252

Buckley, R. M., Davis, B. W., Brashear, W. A., Farias, F. H. G., Kuroki, K., Graves, T., Hillier, L., et al. (2020). A new domestic cat genome assembly based on long sequence reads empowers feline genomic medicine and identifies a novel gene for dwarfism. *PLOS Genetics*,

16(10), e1008926. doi:10.1371/journal.pgen.1008926. https://journals.plos.org/plosgenetics/article?id=10.1371/journal.pgen.1008926

Buscail, E., Alix-Panabières, C., Quincy, P., Cauvin, T., Chauvet, A., Degrandi, O., Caumont, C., et al. (2019). High Clinical Value of Liquid Biopsy to Detect Circulating Tumor Cells and Tumor Exosomes in Pancreatic Ductal Adenocarcinoma Patients Eligible for Up-Front Surgery. *Multidisciplinary Digital Publishing Institute/Cancers*, 11(11). doi:10.3390/cancers11111656. https://www.mdpi.com/2072-6694/11/11/1656

Buscail, L. (2017). Commentary: Pancreatic cancer: is the worst to come? *International Journal of Epidemiology*, 46(6), 1774-1775. doi:10.1093/ije/dyx143. https://academic.oup.com/ije/article/46/6/1774/4082625

Centers for Disease Control and Prevention. (2020, 2016-10-26). National Environmental Public Health Tracking: Pancreatic Cancer. Retrieved from https://ephtracking.cdc.gov/showPancreaticCancer.action

Ceyhan-Birsoy, O., Machini, K., Lebo, M. S., Yu, T. W., Agrawal, P. B., Parad, R. B., Holm, I., et al. (2017). A curated gene list for reporting results of newborn genomic sequencing. *Genetics in Medicine*, 19(7), 809-818. doi:10.1038/gim.2016.193. https://www.nature.com/articles/gim2016193

Ceyhan-Birsoy, O., Murry, J. B., Machini, K., Lebo, M. S., Yu, T. W., Fayer, S., Genetti, C., et al. (2019). Interpretation of Genomic Sequencing Results in Healthy and Ill Newborns: Results from the BabySeq Project. *The American Journal of Human Genetics*, 104(1), 76-93.

doi:10.1016/j.ajhg.2018.11.016.
https://pubmed.ncbi.nlm.nih.gov/30609409/

Cohen, J. D., Li, L., Wang, Y., Thoburn, C., Afsari, B., Danilova, L., Douville, C., et al. (2018). Detection and localization of surgically resectable cancers with a multi-analyte blood test. Science, 359(6378), 926-930. doi:10.1126/science.aar3247. https://science.sciencemag.org/content/359/6378/926

Dockser Marcus, A. (2020, December 9, 2020). Gene Therapy Shows Promise for a Form of Blindness, but Is It a Cure? *The Wall Street Journal.* Retrieved from https://www.wsj.com/articles/gene-therapy-shows-promise-for-a-form-of-blindness-but-is-it-a-cure-11607540844

Expecting Health. (2020). Conditions Screened By State. *Baby's First Test.* Retrieved from https://www.babysfirsttest.org/newborn-screening/states

Fox, M., Galante, A., Lynch, K. (2019). Genetic screening for newborns yields some answers, more questions. *NBC News.* Retrieved from https://www.nbcnews.com/health/health-news/genetic-screening-newborns-yields-some-answers-more-questions-n954511

Franceschini, D., Rossi, S., Loi, M., Chiola, I., Piccoli, F., Lutman, F. R., Finocchiaro, G., Toschi, L., Santoro, A., Scorsetti, M. (2020). Lung cancer management: monitoring and treating resistance development in third-generation EGFR TKIs. *Expert Review of Anticancer Therapy,* 1-11. doi:10.1080/14737140.2020.1806716. https://www.tandfonline.com/doi/abs/10.1080/1473714 0.2020.1806716?journalCode=iery20

Heslop-Harrison, J. S., Schwarzacher, T. (2007).
Domestication, Genomics and the Future for Banana.
Annals of Botany, 100(5), 1073-1084.
doi:10.1093/aob/mcm191.
https://academic.oup.com/aob/article/100/5/1073/137
119

Hofman, P., Heeke, S., Alix-Panabières, C., Pantel, K.
(2019). Liquid biopsy in the era of immuno-oncology: is it
ready for prime-time use for cancer patients? *Annals of
Oncology*, 30(9), 1448-1459. doi:10.1093/annonc/mdz196.
https://www.annalsofoncology.org/article/S0923-
7534(19)45987-5/abstract

Holm, I. A., McGuire, A., Pereira, S., Rehm, H., Green,
R. C., Beggs, A. H. (2019). Returning a Genomic Result
for an Adult-Onset Condition to the Parents of a
Newborn: Insights From the BabySeq Project. *Pediatrics*,
143(Suppl 1), S37-s43. doi:10.1542/peds.2018-1099H.
https://pediatrics.aappublications.org/content/143/Supp
lement_1/S37

Lander, E. S., Linton, L. M., Birren, B., Nusbaum, C.,
Zody, M. C., Baldwin, J., Devon, K., et al. (2001). Initial
sequencing and analysis of the human genome. *Nature*,
409(6822), 860-921. doi:10.1038/35057062.
https://www.nature.com/articles/35057062#Sec1

Le, D. T., Durham, J. N., Smith, K. N., Wang, H.,
Bartlett, B. R., Aulakh, L. K., Lu. S., et al. (2017).
Mismatch repair deficiency predicts response of solid
tumors to PD-1 blockade. *Science*, 357(6349), 409-413.
doi:10.1126/science.aan6733.
https://science.sciencemag.org/content/357/6349/409

Lennon, A. M., Buchanan, A. H., Kinde, I., Warren, A.,
Honushefsky, A., Cohain, A. T., Ledbetter, D. H., et al.
(2020). Feasibility of blood testing combined with PET-

CT to screen for cancer and guide intervention. *Science*, 369(6499). doi:10.1126/science.abb9601. https://science.sciencemag.org/content/369/6499/eabb 9601

Meyer, U. A. (2004). Pharmacogenetics—five decades of therapeutic lessons from genetic diversity. *Nature Reviews: Genetics*, 5(9), 669-676. doi:10.1038/nrg1428. https://www.nature.com/articles/nrg1428

National Cancer Institute, Surveillance, Epidemiology, and End Results Program. (2020). Cancer Stat Facts: Pancreatic Cancer. Retrieved from https://seer.cancer.gov/statfacts/html/pancreas.html

National Human Genome Research Institute. (November 8, 2012). An Overview of the Human Genome Project. Retrieved 2020 from https://www.genome.gov/12011239/a-brief-history-of-the-human-genome-project/

National Human Genome Research Institute. (February 24, 2020). Human Genome Project FAQ. Retrieved 2020 from https://www.genome.gov/human-genome-project/Completion-FAQ

National Human Genome Research Institute. (February 13, 2018). Canine Genome Summary. Retrieved 2020 from https://research.nhgri.nih.gov/dog_genome/canine_gen ome.shtml

National Human Genome Research Institute. (October 11, 2019). What's a Genome? Retrieved 2020 from https://www.genome.gov/About-Genomics/Introduction-to-Genomics#one

Eunice Kennedy Shriver National Institute of Child Health and Human Development. (December 1, 2016). Phenylketonuria (PKU). Retrieved 2020 from https://www.nichd.nih.gov/health/topics/pku

The Nobel Prize. The Nobel Prize in Physiology or Medicine 1962. Retrieved 2020 from https://www.nobelprize.org/prizes/medicine/1962/award-video/#:~:text=The%20Nobel%20Prize%20in%20Physiology%20or%20Medicine%201962%20was%20awarded,information%20transfer%20in%20living%20material.%22

The Nobel Prize. The Nobel Prize in Chemistry 2020. Retrieved 2021 from https://www.nobelprize.org/prizes/chemistry/2020/summary/

Pereira, S., Robinson, J. O., Gutierrez, A. M., Petersen, D. K., Hsu, R. L., Lee, C. H., Schwartz, T. S., et al. (2019). Perceived Benefits, Risks, and Utility of Newborn Genomic Sequencing in the BabySeq Project. *Pediatrics*, 143(Suppl 1), S6-s13. doi:10.1542/peds.2018-1099C. https://pediatrics.aappublications.org/content/143/Supplement_1/S6

Pertea, M., Salzberg, S. L. (2010). Between a chicken and a grape: estimating the number of human genes. Genome biology, 11(5), 206-206. doi:10.1186/gb-2010-11-5-206. https://genomebiology.biomedcentral.com/articles/10.1186/gb-2010-11-5-206

Petrikin, J. E., Cakici, J. A., Clark, M. M., Willig, L. K., Sweeney, N. M., Farrow, E. G., Saunders, C. J., et al. (2018). The NSIGHT1-randomized controlled trial: rapid whole-genome sequencing for accelerated etiologic diagnosis in critically ill infants. *NPJ Genomic Medicine*, 3, 6.

doi:10.1038/s41525-018-0045-8.
https://www.nature.com/articles/s41525-018-0045-8

Ponti, G., Maccaferri, M., Percesepe, A., Tomasi, A., Ozben, T. (2020). Liquid biopsy with cell free DNA: new horizons for prostate cancer. *Critical Reviews in Clinical Laboratory Sciences*, 1-17.
doi:10.1080/10408363.2020.1803789.
https://www.tandfonline.com/doi/abs/10.1080/104083 63.2020.1803789?journalCode=ilab20

Rady Children's Institute for Genomic Medicine. (2020). Rady Children's Shows Genomic Sequencing for Infants in Intensive Care Yields Life-Changing Benefits and Medical Cost Savings [Press release]. Retrieved from https://www.prnewswire.com/news-releases/rady-childrens-shows-genomic-sequencing-for-infants-in-intensive-care-yields-life-changing-benefits-and-medical-cost-savings-301079272.html

Regalado, A. (2020). China's BGI says it can sequence a genome for just $100. *MIT Technology Review*. Retrieved from
https://www.technologyreview.com/2020/02/26/90565 8/china-bgi-100-dollar-genome/

Salkin, A. (September 12, 2008). When in Doubt, Spit It Out. *The New York Times*. Retrieved from https://www.nytimes.com/2008/09/14/fashion/14spit.h tml

Shyamala, K., Girish, H. C., Murgod, S. (2014). Risk of tumor cell seeding through biopsy and aspiration cytology. *Journal of International Society of Preventive & Community Dentistry*, 4(1), 5-11. doi:10.4103/2231-0762.129446.
https://www.ncbi.nlm.nih.gov/pmc/articles/PMC40151 62/

Stadtmauer, E. A., Fraietta, J. A., Davis, M. M., Cohen, A. D., Weber, K. L., Lancaster, E., Mangan, P., et al. (2020). CRISPR-engineered T cells in patients with refractory cancer. *Science*, 367(6481). doi:10.1126/science.aba7365. https://science.sciencemag.org/content/367/6481/eaba7365

Stein, R. (2019). In a 1st, Doctors in US Use CRISPR Tool to Treat Patient with Genetic Disorder. *NPR*. Retrieved from https://www.npr.org/sections/health-shots/2019/07/29/744826505/sickle-cell-patient-reveals-why-she-is-volunteering-for-landmark-gene-editing-st

Stein, R. (2020). A Year In, 1st Patient to Get Gene Editing for Sickle Cell Disease Is Thriving. *NPR*. Retrieved from https://www.npr.org/sections/health-shots/2020/06/23/877543610/a-year-in-1st-patient-to-get-gene-editing-for-sickle-cell-disease-is-thriving

Stein, R. (2020). In a 1st, Scientists Use Revolutionary Gene-Editing Tool to Edit Inside a Patient. *NPR*. Retrieved from https://www.npr.org/sections/health-shots/2020/03/04/811461486/in-a-1st-scientists-use-revolutionary-gene-editing-tool-to-edit-inside-a-patient

Storm, A. C., Lee, L. S. (2016). Endoscopic ultrasound-guided techniques for diagnosing pancreatic mass lesions: Can we do better? *World Journal of Gastroenterology*, 22(39), 8658-8669. doi:10.3748/wjg.v22.i39.8658. https://www.wjgnet.com/1007-9327/full/v22/i39/WJG-22-8658-g003.htm

Tang, K., Gardner, S., Snuderl, M. (2020). The Role of Liquid Biopsies in Pediatric Brain Tumors. *Journal of Neuropathology and Experimental Neurology*, 79(9), 934-940. doi:10.1093/jnen/nlaa068. https://academic.oup.com/jnen/article-abstract/79/9/934/5882050?redirectedFrom=fulltext

US National Library of Medicine. (October 18, 2018).
Rett syndrome. *MedlinePlus*. Retrieved 2020 from
https://medlineplus.gov/ency/article/001536.htm

US National Library of Medicine. (August 17, 2020).
Leber congenital amaurosis. Retrieved from
https://ghr.nlm.nih.gov/condition/leber-congenital-
amaurosis#genes

US Department of Health and Human Services, U. D. o.
E., ;. (1990). Understanding our Genetic Inheritance, The
US Human Genome Project: The First Five Years, Fiscal
Years 1991–1995 (DOE/ER-0452P). Retrieved from
http://www.ornl.gov/sci/techresources/Human_Genom
e/project/5yrplan/summary.shtml

Van Driest, S. L., Shi, Y., Bowton, E. A., Schildcrout, J.
S., Peterson, J. F., Pulley, J., Roden, D. M. (2014).
Clinically actionable genotypes among 10,000 patients
with preemptive pharmacogenomic testing. *Clinical
Pharmacology and Therapeutics*, 95(4), 423-431.
doi:10.1038/clpt.2013.229.
https://ascpt.onlinelibrary.wiley.com/doi/abs/10.1038/c
lpt.2013.229

Venter, J. C., et al., (2001). The Sequence of the Human
Genome. Science, 291(5507), 1304-1351.
doi:10.1126/science.1058040.
https://science.sciencemag.org/content/291/5507/1304

Zhu, Y., Zhang, H., Chen, N., Hao, J., Jin, H., Ma, X.
(2020). Diagnostic value of various liquid biopsy methods
for pancreatic cancer: A systematic review and meta-
analysis. *Medicine*, 99(3), e18581-e18581.
doi:10.1097/MD.0000000000018581.
https://journals.lww.com/md-
journal/Fulltext/2020/01170/Diagnostic_value_of_vario
us_liquid_biopsy_methods.7.aspx

Chapter Six

American Cancer Society. (2021). Global Cancer Facts &
Figures. Retrieved from
https://www.cancer.org/research/cancer-facts-
statistics/global.html

Arcadu, F., Benmansour, F., Maunz, A., Willis, J.,
Haskova, Z., Prunotto, M. (2019). Deep learning
algorithm predicts diabetic retinopathy progression in
individual patients. *npj Digital Medicine*, 2(1), 92.
doi:10.1038/s41746-019-0172-3.
https://www.nature.com/articles/s41746-020-00365-5

Charlson, M. E., Pompei, P., Ales, K. L., MacKenzie, C.
R. (1987). A new method of classifying prognostic
comorbidity in longitudinal studies: development and
validation. *Journal of Clinical Epidemiology*, 40(5), 373-383.
doi:10.1016/0021-9681(87)90171-8.
https://www.jclinepi.com/article/0021-9681(87)90171-
8/fulltext

Chatterjee, N. A., Singh, J. P. (2015). Cardiac
resynchronization therapy: past, present, and future. *Heart
Failure Clinics*, 11(2), 287-303.
doi:10.1016/j.hfc.2014.12.007.
https://pubmed.ncbi.nlm.nih.gov/25834976/

Choi, J., Kwon, L-N., Lim, H., Chun, H-W. (2020).
Gender-Based Analysis of Risk Factors for Dementia
Using Senior Cohort. *International Journal of Environmental
Research and Public Health*, 17(19).
doi:10.3390/ijerph17197274.
https://www.mdpi.com/1660-4601/17/19/7274

Cleveland Clinic. (2021). Heart Failure: Understanding
Heart Failure. Retrieved from
https://my.clevelandclinic.org/health/diseases/17069-

heart-failure-understanding-heart-failure/management-and-treatment

Dontchos, B. N., Yala, A., Barzilay, R., Xiang, J., Lehman, C. D. (2020). External Validation of a Deep Learning Model for Predicting Mammographic Breast Density in Routine Clinical Practice. *Academic Radiology.* doi:10.1016/j.acra.2019.12.012. https://www.academicradiology.org/article/S1076-6332(19)30626-9/abstract

Gao, Y., Sengupta, A., Li, M., Zu, Z., Rogers, B. P., Anderson, A. W., Ding, Z., Gore, J. C. (2020). Functional connectivity of white matter as a biomarker of cognitive decline in Alzheimer's disease. *PLOS One*, 15(10), e0240513. doi:10.1371/journal.pone.0240513. https://journals.plos.org/plosone/article?id=10.1371/journal.pone.0240513

Hu, S-Y., Santus, E., Forsyth, A. W., Malhotra, D., Haimson, J., Chatterjee, N. A., Kramer, D. B., Barzilay, R., Tulsky, J. A., Lindvall, C. (2019). Can machine learning improve patient selection for cardiac resynchronization therapy? *PLOS One*, 14(10), e0222397. doi:10.1371/journal.pone.0222397. https://journals.plos.org/plosone/article?id=10.1371/journal.pone.0222397

Jing, L., Ulloa Cerna, A. E., Good, C. W., Sauers, N. M., Schneider, G., Hartzel, D. N., Leader, J. B., et al. (2020). A Machine Learning Approach to Management of Heart Failure Populations. *JACC: Heart Failure*, 8(7), 578-587. doi:10.1016/j.jchf.2020.01.012. https://www.sciencedirect.com/science/article/abs/pii/S2213177920301384

Levy, W. C., Mozaffarian, D., Linker, D. T., Sutradhar, S. C., Anker, S. D., Cropp, A. B., Anand, I., et al. (2006).

The Seattle Heart Failure Model: prediction of survival in heart failure. *Circulation*, 113(11), 1424-1433. doi:10.1161/circulationaha.105.584102.
https://www.ahajournals.org/doi/10.1161/circulationaha.105.584102

Lin, C-H., Chiu, S-I., Chen, T-F., Jang, J-S. R., Chiu, M-J. (2020). Classifications of Neurodegenerative Disorders Using a Multiplex Blood Biomarkers-Based Machine Learning Model. *International Journal of Molecular Sciences*, 21(18). doi:10.3390/ijms21186914.
https://www.mdpi.com/1422-0067/21/18/6914

Murtagh, P., Greene, G., O'Brien, C. (2020). Current applications of machine learning in the screening and diagnosis of glaucoma: a systematic review and Meta-analysis. *International Journal of Ophthalmology*, 13(1), 149-162. doi:10.18240/ijo.2020.01.22.
https://pubmed.ncbi.nlm.nih.gov/31956584/

National Eye Institute. (November 19, 2020). Diabetic Retinopathy Data and Statistics. Retrieved 2021 from https://www.nei.nih.gov/learn-about-eye-health/resources-for-health-educators/eye-health-data-and-statistics/diabetic-retinopathy-data-and-statistics

Nielsen, K. B., Lautrup, M. L., Andersen, J. K. H., Savarimuthu, T. R., Grauslund, J. (2019). Deep Learning-Based Algorithms in Screening of Diabetic Retinopathy: A Systematic Review of Diagnostic Performance. Ophthalmology Retina, 3(4), 294-304. doi:10.1016/j.oret.2018.10.014.
https://www.ophthalmologyretina.org/article/S2468-6530(18)30487-1/pdf

Raghunath, S., Ulloa Cerna, A. E., Jing, L., vanMaanen, D. P., Stough, J., Hartzel, D. N., Leader, J. B., et al. (2020). Prediction of mortality from 12-lead electrocardiogram voltage data using a deep neural network. *Nature Medicine*, 26(6), 886-891. doi:10.1038/s41591-020-0870-z. https://www.nature.com/articles/s41591-020-0870-z

Rudin, C., Rudin, J. (2019). Why are we using black box models in AI when we don't need to? A lesson from an explainable AI competition. *Harvard Data Science Review*, 1(2). doi: 10.1162/99608f92.5a8a3a3d. https://hdsr.mitpress.mit.edu/pub/f9kuryi8/release/6

Virani, S. S., Alonso, A., Benjamin, E. J., Bittencourt, M. S., Callaway, C. W., Carson, A. P., Chamberlain, A. M., et al., (2020). Heart Disease and Stroke Statistics–2020 Update: A Report From the American Heart Association. *Circulation*, 141(9), e139-e596. doi:10.1161/cir.0000000000000757. https://www.ahajournals.org/doi/10.1161/CIR.0000000000000757

Weng, S. F., Reps, J., Kai, J., Garibaldi, J. M., Qureshi, N. (2017). Can machine-learning improve cardiovascular risk prediction using routine clinical data? *PLOS One*, 12(4), e0174944. doi:10.1371/journal.pone.0174944. https://journals.plos.org/plosone/article?id=10.1371/journal.pone.0174944

World Health Organization. (September 21, 2020). Dementia. Retrieved from https://www.who.int/news-room/fact-sheets/detail/dementia

Yala, A., Lehman, C., Schuster, T., Portnoi, T., Barzilay, R. (2019). A Deep Learning Mammography-based Model for Improved Breast Cancer Risk Prediction. *Radiology*, 292(1), 60-66. doi:10.1148/radiol.2019182716. https://pubs.rsna.org/doi/full/10.1148/radiol.2019182716

Yan, Q., Weeks, D. E., Xin, H., Swaroop, A., Chew, E. Y., Huang, H., Ding, Y., Chen, W. (2020). Deep-learning-based prediction of late age-related macular degeneration progression. *Nature Machine Intelligence*, 2(2), 141-150. doi:10.1038/s42256-020-0154-9. https://www.nature.com/articles/s42256-020-0154-9

Chapter Seven

Bellamy III, W. (2018). Boeing CEO Talks 'Digital Twin' Era of Aviation. *Aviation Today*. Retrieved from https://www.aviationtoday.com/2018/09/14/boeing-ceo-talks-digital-twin-era-aviation/

Belluck, P. (June 21, 2018). A Common Virus May Play Role in Alzheimer's Disease, Study Finds. *The New York Times*. Retrieved from https://www.nytimes.com/2018/06/21/health/alzheimers-virus-herpes.html

Cummings, J., Lee, G., Ritter, A., Sabbagh, M., Zhong, K. (2020). Alzheimer's disease drug development pipeline: 2020. *Alzheimer's Association*, 6(1), e12050. doi:10.1002/trc2.12050. https://alz-journals.onlinelibrary.wiley.com/doi/10.1002/trc2.12050

DiMasi, J. A., Grabowski, H. G., Hansen, R. W. (2016). Innovation in the pharmaceutical industry: New estimates of R&D costs. *Journal of Health Economics*, 47, 20-33. doi:10.1016/j.jhealeco.2016.01.012. https://www.sciencedirect.com/science/article/abs/pii/S0167629616000291

Emerging Technology from the arXiv. (2014). fMRI Data Reveals the Number of Parallel Processes Running in the Brain. *MIT Technology Review*. Retrieved from

https://www.technologyreview.com/2014/11/05/17051
7/fmri-data-reveals-the-number-of-parallel-processes-
running-in-the-brain/

Gerlovin, L., Brooke, B.; Kambo, I.; Ricciardi, G. (2020).
The Expanding Role of Artificial Intelligence in Clinical
Research. *Clinical Leader.* Retrieved from
https://www.clinicalleader.com/doc/the-expanding-role-
of-artificial-intelligence-in-clinical-research-0001

(2021). Charles Fisher on Using Digital Twins to Speed
Clinical Trials. Retrieved from
https://glorikian.com/charles-fisher-on-using-digital-
twins-to-speed-clinical-trials/

(2020). Andrew A. Radin with Progress Report on
TwoXar. Retrieved from https://glorikian.com/andrew-
a-radin-returns-with-a-progress-report-on-twoxar/

Hamilton, J. (2020). Alzheimer's Researchers Go Back to
Basics To Find The Best Way Forward. *NPR.* Retrieved
from https://www.npr.org/sections/health-
shots/2020/06/25/883026917/alzheimer-s-research-is-
going-back-to-basics-to-find-best-way-forward

Arshadi, A. K., Webb, J., Salem, M., Cruz, E., Calad-
Thomson, S., Ghadirian, N., Collins, J., et al. (2020).
Artificial Intelligence for COVID-19 Drug Discovery and
Vaccine Development. *Frontiers in Artificial Intelligence,*
3(65). doi:10.3389/frai.2020.00065.
https://www.frontiersin.org/articles/10.3389/frai.2020.0
0065/full

Kunnumakkara, A. B., Bordoloi, D., Sailo, B. L., Roy, N.
K., Thakur, K. K., Banik, K., Shakibaei, M., Gupta, S. C.,
Aggarwal, B. B. (2019). Cancer drug development: The
missing links. Experimental Biology and Medicine, 244(8),

663-689. doi:10.1177/1535370219839163.
https://pubmed.ncbi.nlm.nih.gov/30961357/

Readhead, B., Haure-Mirande, J. V., Funk, C. C., Richards, M. A., Shannon, P., Haroutunian, V., Sano, M., et al. (2018). Multiscale Analysis of Independent Alzheimer's Cohorts Finds Disruption of Molecular, Genetic, and Clinical Networks by Human Herpesvirus. *Neuron.* doi:10.1016/j.neuron.2018.05.023.
https://pubmed.ncbi.nlm.nih.gov/29937276/

Silipo, R., Widmann, M. (2019). 3 New Techniques for Data-Dimensionality Reduction in Machine Learning. *The New Stack.* Retrieved from https://thenewstack.io/3-new-techniques-for-data-dimensionality-reduction-in-machine-learning/

Stokes, J. M., Yang, K., Swanson, K., Jin, W., Cubillos-Ruiz, A., Donghia, N. M., MacNair, C. R., et al. (2020). A Deep Learning Approach to Antibiotic Discovery. *Cell,* 180(4), 688-702.e613. doi:10.1016/j.cell.2020.01.021.
https://pubmed.ncbi.nlm.nih.gov/32084340/

twoXar Pharmaceuticals. (2021). twoXar Pharmaceuticals Presents Preclinical Data Showing Significant Efficacy and Safety of Two Novel Chronic Kidney Disease Treatment Candidates [Press release]. *Cision PR Newswire.* Retrieved from https://www.prnewswire.com/news-releases/twoxar-pharmaceuticals-presents-preclinical-data-showing-significant-efficacy-and-safety-of-two-novel-chronic-kidney-disease-treatment-candidates-301240747.html

Wang, Y., Li, F., Bharathwaj, M., Rosas, N. C., Leier, A., Akutsu, T., Webb, G. I., et al. (2020). DeepBL: a deep learning-based approach for in silico discovery of beta-lactamases. *Briefings in Bioinformatics.*

doi:10.1093/bib/bbaa301.
https://pubmed.ncbi.nlm.nih.gov/33212503/

Wong, C. H., Siah, K. W., Lo, A. W. (2019). Estimation of clinical trial success rates and related parameters. *Biostatistics*, 20(2), 273-286. doi:10.1093/biostatistics/kxx069. https://academic.oup.com/biostatistics/article/20/2/273/4817524

Chapter Eight

Abdulaal, A., Patel, A., Charani, E., Denny, S., Mughal, N., Moore, L. (2020). Prognostic Modeling of COVID-19 Using Artificial Intelligence in the United Kingdom: Model Development and Validation. *Journal of Medical Internet Research*, 22(8), e20259. doi:10.2196/20259. https://www.jmir.org/2020/8/e20259/

Ackerman, E. (2020). Autonomous Robots Are Helping Kill Coronavirus in Hospitals. *IEEE Spectrum*. Retrieved from https://spectrum.ieee.org/automaton/robotics/medical-robots/autonomous-robots-are-helping-kill-coronavirus-in-hospitals

Apple. (2020). Apple releases new COVID-19 app and website based on CDC guidance [Press release]. Retrieved from https://www.apple.com/newsroom/2020/03/apple-releases-new-covid-19-app-and-website-based-on-CDC-guidance/

Basavaraju, S. V., Patton, M. E., Grimm, K., Rasheed, M. A. U., Lester, S., Mills, L., Stumpf, M., et al. (2020). Serologic testing of US blood donations to identify

SARS-CoV-2-reactive antibodies: December 2019-
January 2020. *Clinical Infectious Diseases.*
doi:10.1093/cid/ciaa1785.
https://academic.oup.com/cid/advance-
article/doi/10.1093/cid/ciaa1785/6012472

Beaubien, J. (2020). More Companies Are Using
Technology To Monitor For Coronavirus In The
Workplace. Retrieved from
https://www.npr.org/2020/10/13/918315238/more-
companies-are-using-technology-to-monitor-for-
coronavirus-in-the-workplace

Bent, B., Dunn, J. P. (2020). Wearables in the SARS-CoV-
2 Pandemic: What Are They Good for? *JMIR Mhealth
Uhealth*, 8(12), e25137. doi:10.2196/25137.
https://mhealth.jmir.org/2020/12/e25137/

Branswell, H. (2020). Chinese scientists obtain genetic
sequence of mysterious virus, a key in containment
efforts. *STAT*. Retrieved from
https://www.statnews.com/2020/01/09/chinese-
scientists-obtain-genetic-sequence-of-mysterious-virus-a-
key-step-in-containment-efforts/

Callaghan, T., Moghtaderi, A., Lueck, J. A., Hotez, P.,
Strych, U., Dor, A., Fowler, E. F., Motta, M. (2021).
Correlates and disparities of intention to vaccinate against
COVID-19. *Social Science & Medicine*, 113638.
doi:https://doi.org/10.1016/j.socscimed.2020.113638.
https://pubmed.ncbi.nlm.nih.gov/33414032/

Centers for Disease Control and Prevention. (December
18, 2020; update March 4, 2021). Understanding mRNA
COVID-19 Vaccines. Retrieved from
https://www.cdc.gov/coronavirus/2019-
ncov/vaccines/different-vaccines/mrna.html

Chen, H., Zhang, Z., Wang, L., Huang, Z., Gong, F., Li, X., Chen, Y., Wu, J. J. (2020). First clinical study using HCV protease inhibitor danoprevir to treat COVID-19 patients. Medicine (Baltimore), 99(48), e23357. doi:10.1097/md.0000000000023357. https://journals.lww.com/md-journal/fulltext/2020/11250/first_clinical_study_using_hcv_protease_inhibitor.53.aspx

Collins, F. (2020). Exploring Drug Repurposing for COVID-19 Treatment. *NIH Director's Blog*. Retrieved from https://directorsblog.nih.gov/tag/leprosy/

Dickson, B. (2020). Why AI might be the most effective weapon we have to fight COVID-19. *Neural*. Retrieved from https://thenextweb.com/neural/2020/03/21/why-ai-might-be-the-most-effective-weapon-we-have-to-fight-covid-19/

Egan, M. (2020). Walmart is using drones to deliver Covid-19 tests. *CNN Business*. Retrieved from https://www.cnn.com/2020/09/23/business/covid-test-drone-delivery-walmart/index.html

Forna, A., Nouvellet, P., Dorigatti, I., Donnelly, C. A. (2020). Case Fatality Ratio Estimates for the 2013-2016 West African Ebola Epidemic: Application of Boosted Regression Trees for Imputation. *Clinical Infectious Diseases*, 70(12), 2476-2483. doi:10.1093/cid/ciz678. https://academic.oup.com/cid/article/70/12/2476/5536742

Giuliano, C., Patel, C. R., Kale-Pradhan, P. B. (2019). A Guide to Bacterial Culture Identification And Results Interpretation. P & T : a peer-reviewed journal for formulary management, 44(4), 192-200. *P & T*. Retrieved from https://pubmed.ncbi.nlm.nih.gov/30930604

Hamel, L., Kirzinger, A., Muñana, C., Brodie, M. (2020). KFF COVID-19 Vaccine Monitor: December 2020. Retrieved from https://www.kff.org/coronavirus-covid-19/report/kff-covid-19-vaccine-monitor-december-2020/

Hassaniazad, M., Bazram, A., Hassanipour, S., Fathalipour, M. (2020). Evaluation of the efficacy and safety of favipiravir and interferon compared to lopinavir/ritonavir and interferon in moderately ill patients with COVID-19: a structured summary of a study protocol for a randomized controlled trial. *Trials*, 21(1), 886. doi:10.1186/s13063-020-04747-8. https://trialsjournal.biomedcentral.com/articles/10.1186/s13063-020-04747-8

Hirten, R. P., Danieletto, M., Tomalin, L., Choi, K. H., Zweig, M., Golden, E., Kaur, S, et al.. (2021). Use of Physiological Data From a Wearable Device to Identify SARS-CoV-2 Infection and Symptoms and Predict COVID-19 Diagnosis: Observational Study. *Journal of Medical Internet Research*, 23(2), e26107. doi:10.2196/26107. https://www.jmir.org/2021/2/e26107/

Holshue, M. L., DeBolt, C., Lindquist, S., Lofy, K. H., Wiesman, J., Bruce, H., Spitters, C., et al. (2020). First Case of 2019 Novel Coronavirus in the United States. *New England Journal of Medicine*, 382(10), 929-936. doi:10.1056/NEJMoa2001191. https://www.nejm.org/doi/full/10.1056/NEJMoa2001191

Keni, R., Alexander, A., Nayak, P. G., Mudgal, J., Nandakumar, K. (2020). COVID-19: Emergence, Spread, Possible Treatments, and Global Burden. *Frontiers in Public Health*, 8(216). doi:10.3389/fpubh.2020.00216. https://www.frontiersin.org/articles/10.3389/fpubh.2020.00216/full

Kent, J. (2020). New Initiative Uses Artificial Intelligence for Vaccine Development. *Health IT Analytics*. Retrieved from https://healthitanalytics.com/news/new-initiative-uses-artificial-intelligence-for-vaccine-development

Kurzweil, R. (2020). AI-Powered Biotech Can Help Deploy a Vaccine In Record Time. *Wired*. Retrieved from https://www.wired.com/story/opinion-ai-powered-biotech-can-help-deploy-a-vaccine-in-record-time/

Laguarta, J., Hueto, F., Subirana, B. (2020). COVID-19 Artificial Intelligence Diagnosis Using Only Cough Recordings. *IEEE Open Journal of Engineering in Medicine and Biology*, 1, 275-281. doi:10.1109/OJEMB.2020.3026928. https://ieeexplore.ieee.org/document/9208795

Landi, H. (2020). Boston startup using AI, remote monitoring to fight coronavirus. *Fierce Healthcare*. Retrieved from https://www.fiercehealthcare.com/tech/boston-startup-using-ai-remote-monitoring-to-fight-coronavirus

Miliard, M. (2020). AI models from Mount Sinai can predict critical COVID-19 cases. *Healthcare IT News*. Retrieved from https://www.healthcareitnews.com/news/ai-models-mount-sinai-can-predict-critical-covid-19-cases

Neher, R. A., Bedford, T. (2018). Real-Time Analysis and Visualization of Pathogen Sequence Data. *Journal of Clinical Microbiology*, 56(11), e00480-00418. doi:10.1128/JCM.00480-18. https://pubmed.ncbi.nlm.nih.gov/30135232/

Niiler, E. (2020). An AI Epidemiologist Sent the First Warnings of the Wuhan Virus. *Wired*. Retrieved from https://www.wired.com/story/ai-epidemiologist-wuhan-public-health-warnings/

Orlandic, L., Teijeiro, T., Atienza, D. (2020). The COUGHVID crowdsourcing data set: A corpus for the study of large-scale cough analysis algorithms. *Cornell University/arXiv.org*. Retrieved from https://arxiv.org/abs/2009.11644

Perkins, R. (2020). Students Use AI for a Better COVID-19 Prediction Model. *Caltech*. Retrieved from https://www.caltech.edu/about/news/students-use-ai-better-prediction-covid-19-model

Riva, L., Yuan, S., Yin, X., Martin-Sancho, L., Matsunaga, N., Pache, L., Burgstaller-Muehlbacher, S., et al. (2020). Discovery of SARS-CoV-2 antiviral drugs through large-scale compound repurposing. *Nature*, 586(7827), 113-119. doi:10.1038/s41586-020-2577-1. https://pubmed.ncbi.nlm.nih.gov/32707573/

Saltmarsh, A. (2020). Summit — the Supercomputer Fighting Coronavirus. *Direct Indusry e-mag*. Retrieved from http://emag.directindustry.com/summit-the-supercomputer-fighting-coronavirus/

Taubenberger, J. K., Morens, D. M. (2006). 1918 Influenza: the mother of all pandemics. *Emerging Infectious Diseases*, 12(1), 15-22. doi:10.3201/eid1201.050979. https://wwwnc.cdc.gov/eid/article/12/1/05-0979_article

US Food and Drug Administration. (2020). Coronavirus (COVID-19) Update: FDA Issues Emergency Use Authorization for Potential COVID-19 Treatment [Press release]. Retrieved from https://www.fda.gov/news-events/press-announcements/coronavirus-covid-19-

update-fda-issues-emergency-use-authorization-potential-covid-19-treatment

University of California Museum of Paleontology. (2021). Molecular clocks. *Understanding Evolution.* Retrieved from https://evolution.berkeley.edu/evolibrary/article/molecc locks_01

Warren, T. K., Jordan, R., Lo, M. K., Ray, A. S., Mackman, R. L., Soloveva, V., Siegel, D., et al. (2016). Therapeutic efficacy of the small molecule GS-5734 against Ebola virus in rhesus monkeys. *Nature,* 531(7594), 381-385. doi:10.1038/nature17180. https://www.nature.com/articles/nature17180

Yang, Y., Zhu, J. (2020). Coronavirus brings China's surveillance state out of the shadows. *Reuters.* Retrieved from https://www.reuters.com/article/us-china-health-surveillance/coronavirus-brings-chinas-surveillance-state-out-of-the-shadows-idUSKBN2011HO

Chapter Nine

Abrams, R. (2017, May 23, 2017). Target to Pay $18.5 Million to 47 States in Security Breach Settlement. *The New York Times.* Retrieved from https://www.nytimes.com/2017/05/23/business/target-security-breach-settlement.html

Alexander, W. (2013). Barnaby Jack Could Hack Your Pacemaker and Make Your Heart Explode. *Vice.* Retrieved from https://www.vice.com/en/article/avnx5j/i-worked-out-how-to-remotely-weaponise-a-pacemaker

Andrews, E. E., Forber-Pratt, A. J., Mona, L. R., Lund, E. M., Pilarski, C. R., Balter, R. (2019). #SaytheWord: A disability culture commentary on the erasure of "disability". *Rehabilitation Psychology*, 64(2), 111-118. doi:10.1037/rep0000258. https://psycnet.apa.org/doiLanding?doi=10.1037%2Frep0000258

Cavallo, J. (2019). Confronting the Criticisms Facing Watson for Oncology. *The ASCO Post*. Retrieved from https://ascopost.com/issues/september-10-2019/confronting-the-criticisms-facing-watson-for-oncology/

Centers for Disease Control and Prevention, & National Center on Birth Defects and Developmental Disabilities. (June 8, 2020). Data and Statistics About Hearing Loss in Children. Retrieved 2021 from https://www.cdc.gov/ncbddd/hearingloss/data.html

Chien, W. W. (2018). A CRISPR Way to Restore Hearing. *The New England Journal of Medicine*, 378(13), 1255-1256. doi:10.1056/NEJMcibr1716789. https://www.nejm.org/doi/10.1056/NEJMcibr1716789

Cohen, I. G. (2020). Informed Consent and Medical Artificial Intelligence: What to Tell the Patient? *Georgetown Law Journal*, 108, 1425-1469. doi:10.2139/ssrn.3529576. https://www.law.georgetown.edu/georgetown-law-journal/in-print/volume-108-issue-6-june-2020/informed-consent-and-medical-artificial-intelligence-what-to-tell-the-patient/

Davis, J. (2020). UPDATE: The 10 Biggest Healthcare Data Breaches of 2020. *Health IT Security*. Retrieved from https://healthitsecurity.com/news/the-10-biggest-healthcare-data-breaches-of-2020

Evans, B. (2013). How autism became autism: The radical transformation of a central concept of child development in Britain. *History of Human Sciences*, 26(3), 3-31. doi:10.1177/0952695113484320. https://pubmed.ncbi.nlm.nih.gov/24014081/

Gianfrancesco, M. A., Tamang, S., Yazdany, J., Schmajuk, G. (2018). Potential Biases in Machine Learning Algorithms Using Electronic Health Record Data. *JAMA Internal Medicine*, 178(11), 1544-1547. doi:10.1001/jamainternmed.2018.3763. https://jamanetwork.com/journals/jamainternalmedicine/article-abstract/2697394

Glisson, W. B., Andel, T., McDonald, T., Jacobs, M., Campbell, M., Mayr, J. (2015). Compromising a medical mannequin. *Cornell University/arXiv.org*. preprint arXiv:1509.00065. https://arxiv.org/abs/1509.00065

Goh, K. H., Wang, L., Yeow, A. Y. K., Poh, H., Li, K., Yeow, J. J. L., Tan, G. Y. H. (2021). Artificial intelligence in sepsis early prediction and diagnosis using unstructured data in healthcare. *Nature Communications*, 12(1), 711. doi:10.1038/s41467-021-20910-4. https://www.nature.com/articles/s41467-021-20910-4

Gonçalves, L. S., Amaro, M. L. M., Romero, A. L. M., Schamne, F. K., Fressatto, J. L., Bezerra, C. W. (2020). Implementation of an Artificial Intelligence Algorithm for sepsis detection. *Revista Brasileira de Enfermagem*, 73(3), e20180421. doi:10.1590/0034-7167-2018-0421. https://pubmed.ncbi.nlm.nih.gov/32294705/

György, B., Nist-Lund, C., Pan, B., Asai, Y., Karavitaki, K. D., Kleinstiver, B. P., Garcia, S. P., et al. (2019). Allele-specific gene editing prevents deafness in a model of dominant progressive hearing loss. *Nature Medicine*, 25(7),

1123-1130. doi:10.1038/s41591-019-0500-9.
https://pubmed.ncbi.nlm.nih.gov/31270503/

Hart, R. D. (2017). When artificial intelligence botches your medical diagnosis, who's to blame? *Quartz*. Retrieved from https://qz.com/989137/when-a-robot-ai-doctor-misdiagnoses-you-whos-to-blame/

Hodges, H., Fealko, C., Soares, N. (2020). Autism spectrum disorder: definition, epidemiology, causes, and clinical evaluation. *Translational Pediatrics*, 9(Suppl 1), S55-s65. doi:10.21037/tp.2019.09.09.
https://pubmed.ncbi.nlm.nih.gov/32206584/

Jercich, K. (2020). AI bias may worsen COVID-19 health disparities for people of color. *Healthcare IT News*. Retrieved from https://www.healthcareitnews.com/news/ai-bias-may-worsen-covid-19-health-disparities-people-color

Katz, S. (August 11, 2020). Why Deaf People Oppose Using Gene Editing to "Cure" Deafness. *Discover*. Retrieved from https://www.discovermagazine.com/health/why-deaf-people-oppose-using-gene-editing-to-cure-deafness

Kotsopoulos, J. (2018). BRCA Mutations and Breast Cancer Prevention. *Cancers*, 10(12), 524. doi:10.3390/cancers10120524.
https://www.mdpi.com/2072-6694/10/12/524

Landi, H. (2020). Average cost of healthcare data breach rises to $7.1M, according to IBM report. *Fierce Healthcare*. Retrieved from https://www.fiercehealthcare.com/tech/average-cost-healthcare-data-breach-rises-to-7-1m-according-to-ibm-report

Longoni, C., Bonezzi, A., Morewedge, C. K. (2019). Resistance to Medical Artificial Intelligence. *Journal of Consumer Research*, 46(4), 629-650. doi:10.1093/jcr/ucz013. https://academic.oup.com/jcr/article/46/4/629/548529 2

Longoni, C., Morewedge, C. K. (2019). AI Can Outperform Doctors. So Why Don't Patients Trust It? *Harvard Business Review*. Retrieved from https://hbr.org/2019/10/ai-can-outperform-doctors-so-why-dont-patients-trust-it

Luzzatto, L. (2012). Sickle cell anaemia and malaria. *Mediterranean Journal of Hematology and Infectious Diseases*, 4(1), e2012065-e2012065. doi:10.4084/MJHID.2012.065. https://www.mjhid.org/index.php/mjhid/article/view/2 012.065

Michie, M., Allyse, M. (2018). Many Families with Down syndrome Children Would Consider Gene Modification, but with Serious Concerns. *Harvard Law Petrie-Flom Bill of Health*. Retrieved from https://blog.petrieflom.law.harvard.edu/2018/09/27/ma ny-families-with-down-syndrome-children-would-consider-gene-modification-but-with-serious-concerns/

Neergaard, L. (2018). Most Americans support gene-editing embryos to prevent diseases, poll shows. *STAT*. Retrieved from https://www.statnews.com/2018/12/28/poll-americans-support-gene-editing-embryos-to-prevent-disease

Obermeyer, Z., Powers, B., Vogeli, C., Mullainathan, S. (2019). Dissecting racial bias in an algorithm used to manage the health of populations. *Science*, 366(6464), 447-453. doi:10.1126/science.aax2342. https://science.sciencemag.org/content/366/6464/447

Paulus, J. K., Kent, D. M. (2020). Predictably unequal: understanding and addressing concerns that algorithmic clinical prediction may increase health disparities. *Nature: npj Digital Medicine*, 3(1), 99. doi:10.1038/s41746-020-0304-9. https://www.nature.com/articles/s41746-020-0304-9

Pierson, E., Cutler, D. M., Leskovec, J., Mullainathan, S., Obermeyer, Z. (2021). An algorithmic approach to reducing unexplained pain disparities in underserved populations. *Nature: Nature Medicine*, 27(1), 136-140. doi:10.1038/s41591-020-01192-7. https://www.nature.com/articles/s41591-020-01192-7

Regalado, A. (2018). EXCLUSIVE: Chinese scientists are creating CRISPR babies. *MIT Technology Review*. Retrieved from https://www.technologyreview.com/2018/11/25/138962/exclusive-chinese-scientists-are-creating-crispr-babies/

Robbins, R., Brodwin, E. (2020). An invisible hand: Patients aren't being told about the AI systems advising their care. *STAT*. Retrieved from https://www.statnews.com/2020/07/15/artificial-intelligence-patient-consent-hospitals/

Röösli, E., Rice, B., Hernandez-Boussard, T. (2020). Bias at warp speed: how AI may contribute to the disparities gap in the time of COVID-19. *Journal of the American Medical Informatics Association*. doi:10.1093/jamia/ocaa210. https://academic.oup.com/jamia/article/28/1/190/5893483

Ross, C., Swetlitz, I. (2017). IBM pitched its Watson supercomputer as a revolution in cancer care. It's nowhere close. *STAT*. Retrieved from https://www.statnews.com/2017/09/05/watson-ibm-cancer/

Shearer, A. E., Hildebrand, M. S., Smith, R. J. H. (1993; Last update: July 27, 2017). Hereditary Hearing Loss and Deafness Overview. M. P. Adam, H. H. Ardinger, R. A. Pagon, S. E. Wallace, L. J. H. Bean, G. Mirzaa, A. Amemiya (Eds.), *GeneReviews(®) [Internet]*. Seattle (WA): University of Washington, Seattle. Copyright © 1993-2021, University of Washington, Seattle. (GeneReviews is a registered trademark of the University of Washington, Seattle. All rights reserved.) https://www.ncbi.nlm.nih.gov/books/NBK1434/

Swalin, A. (2018). How to Handle Missing Data. *Towards Data Science*. Retrieved from https://towardsdatascience.com/how-to-handle-missing-data-8646b18db0d4

Uzuner, Ö. (2009). Recognizing obesity and comorbidities in sparse data. *Journal of the American Medical Informatics Association*, 16(4), 561-570. doi:10.1197/jamia.M3115. https://academic.oup.com/jamia/article/16/4/561/766997

Wartman, S. A., Combs, C. D. (2019). Reimagining Medical Education in the Age of AI. *AMA Journal of Ethics*, 21(2), E146-152. doi:10.1001/amajethics.2019.146. https://journalofethics.ama-assn.org/article/reimagining-medical-education-age-ai/2019-02

Whelton, P. K., Carey, R. M., Aronow, W. S., Casey Jr., D. E., Collins, K. J., Dennison Himmelfarb, C., DePalma, S. M., et al. (2018). 2017 ACC/AHA/AAPA/ABC/ACPM/AGS/APhA/ASH/ASPC/NMA/PCNA Guideline for the Prevention, Detection, Evaluation, and Management of High Blood Pressure in Adults: A Report of the American College of Cardiology/American Heart Association Task Force on Clinical Practice Guidelines. *Hypertension*, 71(6), e13-e115.

doi:10.1161/hyp.0000000000000065.
https://www.ahajournals.org/doi/full/10.1161/HYP.000
0000000000065

Wynants, L., Van Calster, B., Collins, G. S., Riley, R. D., Heinze, G., Schuit, E., Bonten, M. M. J., et al. (2020). Prediction models for diagnosis and prognosis of covid-19 infection: systematic review and critical appraisal. *BMJ (Clinical Research Ed.)*, 369, m1328. doi:10.1136/bmj.m1328.
https://www.bmj.com/content/369/bmj.m1328

Yuan, K-C., Tsai, L-W., Lee, K-H., Cheng, Y-W., Hsu, S-C., Lo, Y-S., Chen, R-J. (2020). The development an artificial intelligence algorithm for early sepsis diagnosis in the intensive care unit. *International Journal of Medical Informatics*, 141, 104176. doi:
https://doi.org/10.1016/j.ijmedinf.2020.104176

Chapter Ten

Greshko, M. (December 5, 2019). These are the top 20 scientific discoveries of the decade. *National Geographic*. Retrieved from
https://www.nationalgeographic.com/science/2019/12/top-20-scientific-discoveries-of-decade-2010s/

ABOUT THE AUTHOR

For over twenty-five years Harry Glorikian—healthcare entrepreneur, author, podcaster, and company leader—has been at the intersection of the fast-moving science and business of healthcare and biotechnology. Harry has always been at the forefront, helping invest in and grow innovative healthcare companies that are tackling ground-breaking areas such as precision medicine and the human genome. Whether growing and selling his own consulting company, Scientia Advisors, or as an entrepreneur-in-residence at GE Healthcare, or as a general partner at Scientia Ventures, Harry's insatiably curious mind has led him to explore and tackle all sides of healthcare and biotechnology innovation. He has always found himself at the vanguard of cutting-edge technologies in healthcare. His mantra has always been, "We have the opportunity to change the world through better healthcare!" As a recognized thought leader, Harry has spoken at industry conferences and seminars all over the world and is regularly interviewed and quoted by *CBS, ABC, WGBH, Dow Jones, The Boston Globe, BioWorld Today, The Los Angeles Times, The Independent Newspaper London, Medical Device Daily, Science Magazine, Genetic Engineering & Biotechnology News*, and many other media outlets. Harry is the author of *MoneyBall Medicine: Thriving in the New Data-Driven Healthcare Market* and the diagnostics textbook *Commercializing Novel IVDs: A Comprehensive Manual for Success*, and is the host of The Harry Glorikian Show podcast series. In *The Future You*, Harry brings his knowledge and experience to the general consumer who wants to understand how all this new technology and talk of artificial intelligence can make their lives and those of their family and friends more fulfilling through better health.